A Clinician's Guide to Understanding and Using Psychoanalysis in Practice

This book provides an intimate portrait of a clinician's psychoanalytic approach to working in the public health sector with people suffering from acute and chronic emotional pain.

Drawing on three central psychoanalytic concepts of countertransference, projective identification, and the destructive superego, Paul Terry weaves together a unique and distinctive psychoanalytically-based approach to psychotherapeutic work. He illustrates this approach in detailed, almost moment-by-moment case studies of his work with people suffering from depression, psychosis, dependency, loneliness, dementia, and terminal illness. He also shows how his approach helps him to understand social and political issues of war, the holocaust, entitlement, and sexual identity. For readers unfamiliar with psychoanalytic theory, the book concludes with an appendix in which there is a summary of some Kleinian psychoanalytic concepts and psychoanalytic studies of psychosis.

This informative, compelling, and moving book will act as a valuable resource for students training in psychoanalysis and to work in public settings along with career psychologists and mental health professionals seeking to better understand their clients and experiences.

Paul Terry is a Consultant Clinical Psychologist in private practice. During a career in public health spanning four decades Paul has worked in child, adolescent, adult mental health, forensic settings, and latterly in a specialist mental health service for older people. In tandem with clinical practice, he was lecturer in Counselling at Birkbeck College, University of London.

'Paul Terry's unique blend of clarity, rigour, warmth and candour makes this a valuable addition for both experienced and trainee counsellors and psychotherapists. It elucidates key theoretical ideas and detailed clinical processes as well as broadening out to offer intriguing insight into wider political and social issues.'

Sue Kegerreis, *Department of Psychosocial and Psychoanalytic Studies, University of Essex*

A Clinician's Guide to Understanding and Using Psychoanalysis in Practice

Paul Terry

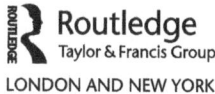
Routledge
Taylor & Francis Group

LONDON AND NEW YORK

Designed cover image: Pobytov, courtesy of Getty Images

First published 2023
by Routledge
4 Park Square, Milton Park, Abingdon, Oxon OX14 4RN

and by Routledge
605 Third Avenue, New York, NY 10158

Routledge is an imprint of the Taylor & Francis Group, an informa business

British Library Cataloguing-in-Publication Data
A catalogue record for this book is available from the British Library

ISBN: 9781032334462 (hbk)
ISBN: 9781032334455 (pbk)
ISBN: 9781003319719 (ebk)

DOI: 10.4324/9781003319719

Typeset in Garamond
by Newgen Publishing UK

To my husband Philip Chklar
for his love

Contents

Acknowledgments

Psychoanalysis has helped me see that the passion and endurance I bring to the therapeutic endeavour reflects the wish to repair my damaged internal objects. In other words, this means acknowledging the importance of my damaged family of origin together with those who have become my family and whose love has helped me develop and sustain the work. This external world to whom I owe my gratitude also includes my colleagues, supervisees, students, and crucially my therapists and supervisors. I am grateful to my patients who have engaged with me in arduous and painful work, challenging and inspiring me.

I would like to express my thanks to Rossana Kendall and Sarah Clarke for their perspicacious comments about early parts of the manuscript for this book, and to Esther Ramsay-Jones who generously offered comments on the entire draft as it neared completion. I am grateful for the most helpful suggestions from the anonymous reviewers of the manuscript. It has been an enormous pleasure collaborating with my editor Grace McDonnell who has brought enthusiasm and wise counsel to our endeavour. I would also like to thank the other members of the Routledge editorial team Georgina Clutterbuck, Helen Evans and Jonathan Merrett who have helped me in the production of this book. I am hugely indebted to William Halton who, many years ago was my first psychoanalytic supervisor. More recently he has mentored much of my writing and latterly contributed greatly to this manuscript. I feel most fortunate to have benefitted from his insight, scholarship and wisdom.

Credits List

The author also gratefully acknowledges permission to republish the following materials:

Paul Terry (2012). Regime change and the superego. *Psychodynamic Practice*, *18* (3), 325–38, DOI: 10.1080/14753634.2012.694219

Paul Terry (2014). Not too late: Fortnightly short term dynamic therapy with older people. *Psychodynamic Practice*, *20* (4), 362–72, DOI: 10.1080/14753634.2014.946953

Paul Terry (2018). Fears of death and fears of dying in the countertransference. *Psychodynamic Practice*, *24* (2), 160–71, DOI: 10.1080/14753634.2018.1458642

Paul Terry (2005). Dangerous liaisons: Psychosis and violence – working in a psychiatric intensive care unit. *Psychoanalytic Psychotherapy*, *19* (3), 221–32, DOI: 10.1080/02668730500238234

Paul Terry (2003). Working with psychosis. *Psychodynamic Practice*, *9* (2), 123–40, DOI: 10.1080/1353333031000104802

Paul Terry (2004). Working with psychosis: Part 2 – Encounters with an omnipotent super-ego. *Psychodynamic Practice*, *10* (1), 45–59, DOI: 10.1080/14753630310001656036

Paul Terry (2005). Working with psychosis: Part 3 – Struggling to contain madness – losing and recovering a capacity to think. *Psychodynamic Practice*, *11* (1), 29–39, DOI: 10.1080/14753630400030106

Paul Terry (2010). Working with psychosis Part 4 – Therapy online – ending by email. *Psychodynamic Practice*, *16* (2), 151–63, DOI: 10.1080/14753631003688126

Paul Terry (2002). A commentary on the film *No Man's Land* for the PPOWP APS Interest Group. *Psychodynamic Practice*, *8* (4), 532–6, DOI: 10.1080/14753630215949

Paul Terry (2014). Beware of pity which conceals envy. *Psychodynamic Practice*, *20* (3), 280–4, DOI: 10.1080/14753634.2014.916842

Paul Terry (2015). On reading *The Uncommon Reader*. *Psychodynamic Practice*, *21* (3), 264–8, DOI: 10.1080/14753634.2015.1036631

Paul Terry (2019). Sexual identity and mourning in the novel *Nora Webster*. *Psychodynamic Practice*, *25* (2), 162–6, DOI: 10.1080/14753634.2018.1557857

Introduction – Projective Identification, Counter-Transference and the Destructive Superego

This guide to using psychoanalysis is a portrait of my approach to helping patients in pain and distress whom I have encountered working as a clinical psychologist. I hope this portrait will help you, the reader, with your approach to therapeutic work. My approach is illustrated by examples from work in various public health settings, including how I needed to manage the organisational realities and demands. The first three parts – which are about Depression, Death and Psychosis – are based on articles[1] about my clinical work. The fourth part, Life, is based on articles[2] using my approach to think about unconscious processes in our social and political world. In the following introduction, I outline the theoretical underpinning of my approach and its implications for therapeutic technique. Firstly, there is an account of the key psychoanalytic concepts which inform my approach, particularly in the way these concepts have developed within the Kleinian school of psychoanalysis. Then there is a discussion of how these concepts have shaped my therapeutic technique. The chapter concludes with summaries about how my approach is illustrated[3] in the four parts of the book.

For readers unfamiliar with Kleinian thought there is a brief summary of some central Kleinian ideas in Appendix 1.

Key Concepts in My Approach: Projective Identification, Counter-transference and the Destructive Superego

Projective Identification

Klein introduced projective identification in her 1946 paper 'Notes on Some Schizoid Mechanisms', in which she formulated the paranoid-schizoid position. Projective identification was a significant development of Freud's understanding of projection. Projective identification has proved enormously influential in psychoanalytic, psychodynamic and other schools of therapy.

Klein understood projective identification to predominate when the mind is beset by persecutory fears and defences in paranoid-schizoid states. Klein

DOI: 10.4324/9781003319719-1

described the mind engaging in an omnipotent unconscious phantasy modelled on bodily function of expelling excrements, in which 'bad' parts of the self could be disowned, split off and projected in phantasy into someone else who is then identified with those parts of the self. Projective identification denies separateness by treating the other as an extension of oneself. Klein added that just as excrements can be felt to be gifts, so 'good' parts of the self can also be projected. She discussed the consequent splitting and depletion of the ego (meaning the self) that resulted from this defence. Projective identification of parts of the self is used in unconscious phantasy to possess and control the internal or external object because bad parts can be felt to be dangerous to the self or because good parts, although felt unmanageable are valuable for the self and not to be lost. The essential elements of projective identification are splitting, denial, projection and identification used in phantasy to possess, control and deny separateness. The recovery and re-integration of these split-off and lost parts of the self, good and bad, is a central element of the therapeutic process.

One of Klein's famous protégés, Wilfrid Bion (1962) elaborated an understanding of how projective identification can be a means of interpersonal communication, beginning early in infancy and used throughout life. When the infant projects unbearable painful states, the success of this as a communication relies on the mother's or primary carer's sensitivity and openness to the infant's emotional states. Bion elaborated the mother's capacity to receive and contain the infant's projections in a 'maternal reverie'. By her love and understanding she can transform the infant's unbearable emotional experiences into something that can be understood. That is to say, as mother comes to know her infant through projective identification, she helps him or her to know him- or herself, to bear emotional pain and eventually use language for thought. Bion proposed maternal containment as a model for the containment a therapist provides for a patient, by virtue of the therapist's sensitivity and receptiveness for the patient's projective identifications. The projections provide a way for the therapist to understand more about the patient, and for enabling the patient in reaching an understanding of him- or herself.

Projective identification is not simply a passive unconscious phantasy of lodging aspects of oneself in someone else. By various subtle, subliminal means in verbal and non-verbal behaviour, for example a tone of voice or a raised eyebrow, the recipients of our projections can be induced to think and feel in a way that is resonant with the projective phantasy. For example, if the patient needs to project an unbearable sadness the therapist may begin to feel a deep sadness, whilst the patient may not appear sad or have conscious awareness of sadness. It is not uncommon for this unconscious communication to be described as the patient concretely putting his or her sadness into the therapist. This way of describing the process is confused with the patient's unconscious phantasy of being able to expel his or her unwanted feeling into the therapist. The sadness the therapist feels is not the patient's sadness, but the therapist's own sadness which has been projectively evoked, usually from an unconscious need for these feelings to be understood. Bion (1962) called this 'realistic projective identification', and more recently Spillius (2012) has suggested the term 'evocative' projective identification. Britton (2003) uses the term 'attributive' projective identification which reflects the Kleinian understanding that corresponding feelings may or may not be evoked in the recipient of the projection. In this book projective identification is used primarily in the Spillius 'evocative' sense, though I will indicate where I believe a different form of projective identification is present.

In one of her few later writings about projective identification Klein published a paper titled 'On Identification' (1955) in which she explored projective identification in relation to a novel *If I were you* by Julian Green (1947). Klein discussed how, in different episodes of the novel, the main character projects his whole self into others in order to take over their identities. This is a different form of projective identification from the original meaning described earlier in the phantasy of expelling parts of the self into others. This form of projective identification is about taking over qualities of others and in its most extreme, as depicted in the novel, means taking over the whole of the other's identity. This form of projective identification has been somewhat overlooked until Britton (2003) suggested it be described as 'acquisitive projective identification'. Joseph (1987) discusses how acquisitive and attributive projective identification can occur simultaneously, and gives clinical illustrations of the simultaneous phantasies of being able to put uncomfortable aspects of oneself into the other at same time as being able to take over desired aspects of the other.

Sodre (2012) has argued that projective identification is an umbrella term which includes projective and introjective identification. Spillius (2012) agrees with Sodre and sees introjective identification as part of acquisitive projective identification. Sodre points out that often introjective identification has been mistakenly thought of as a mature form of identification, because it is a symbolic identification with another which acknowledges separateness, for example in 'I wish I was like the other'. Whereas acquisitive projective identification has been thought of as a concrete form of identification with another, effectively 'I am the other'. Sodre argues both projective and introjective identification may at times be concrete or symbolic. For example in depressive states of mind projective identification is used as the basis of empathy with the other, in a symbolic form of identification which recognises separateness (Joseph, 1987). This can be seen as a form of acquisitive projective identification used as a means of temporarily putting oneself in someone else's shoes as a way of trying to understand that person. The projections are only temporary and are withdrawn out of respect for the integrity of the other.

Counter-transference

Counter-transference refers to the therapist's thoughts, feelings or reverie in the therapeutic encounter. Freud saw the counter-transference as essentially the result of the therapist's transference to the patient, and which could be a matter of concern about the mental state of the therapist. Early in the development of psychoanalysis if therapists introduced their feelings whilst discussing a patient, the tendency was to think it was an indication of the therapist's own problems intruding, and could suggest a need to return to personal therapy. In 1950, Heimann wrote what has become a seminal paper about counter-transference in which she heralded a shift in psychoanalytic thinking from seeing counter-transference as a hindrance to an appreciation of its value. She stressed the importance of therapists not discharging their feelings into action, but instead reflecting on them as a possible source of unconscious communication from the patient. This shift in thinking contributes to the centrality counter-transference has in current psychoanalytic and psychodynamic practice. More recently, thinking about counter-transference has been extended to include monitoring bodily sensations (Lemma, 2014). Hinshelwood (1994) has emphasised the importance of anchoring reflections on the counter-transference in the study of the detail of the clinical material.

In the 1946 paper which introduced projective identification Klein made particular acknowledgment of Paula Heimann's contributions. Although Heimann did not explicitly refer to the concept of projective identification in her paper on counter-transference, it is likely her understanding of projective identification contributed to her insights about counter-transference. Projective identification sheds a light on how the therapist's counter-transference becomes a source of clues about the patient's unconscious communication. This illumination can help therapists in the complex process of disentangling what belongs to the therapist and what belongs to the patient. Reflecting on the counter-transference can be seen as a way of discovering how one's own feelings may be being projectively evoked as an unconscious communication about aspects of the patient's feelings. The unconscious hope in this projective process is that if the therapist can bear those feelings, then perhaps the patient may eventually be able to bear the feelings.

Appreciating the role of projective identification in counter-transference is especially helpful because when our feelings are evoked projectively in the counter-transference we can mistakenly believe our feelings are only about us. Furthermore, Money-Kyrle (1956) acknowledged how disturbing our counter-transference feelings can be. In Brenman-Pick's (1985) paper about the working through of such disturbances she described how patients' projections can be finely attuned to specific, and at times troubling aspects of ourselves, for example the wish to be all-knowing, or to deny one's sadism, or most especially our guilt (p. 161).

We need to be able to bear and remain curious about our feelings, especially those feelings which may be painfully discordant with our views of ourselves, and which we may wish to deny (Steyn, 2013). Thinking about the counter-transference can be obstructed because the projective processes can include persecutory guilt about one's feelings, which evoke what Brenman-Pick described as the therapist's 'superego anxiety'. If we are able to maintain an attitude of curiosity about our struggles, we may come to see how thinking about our feelings can reveal a communication about the patient's struggles and guilt which found a resonance with our own.

The Destructive Superego

Together with projective identification and counter-transference the other key concept in my approach to therapy is that of the destructive superego.

The term superego was first introduced by Freud (1923) in *The Ego and the Id*. He proposed the superego was the 'heir to the Oedipus Complex', formed from a part of the ego which identified with the parents, especially their standards, values and morality. At first, he saw the superego as promoting life and development, whether through setting ideals or through threats of punishment. He saw the superego as the seat of the conscience, in part conscious and in part unconscious, and often the source of unconscious guilt. Later Freud described a more sinister superego which prevented recovery by maintaining it was morally wrong and made patients feel guilty about their emotional difficulties. His studies of depression revealed the influence of what he described as a sadistic superego.

Klein (1958) came to different conclusions about the origin of the superego. It was not based on an internalised identification with the parents or external authorities but arose from an internal conflict within the self:

> In my view, the splitting of the ego, by which the super-ego is formed, comes about as a consequence of conflict in the ego, engendered by the polarity of the two (life and death) instincts. This conflict is increased by their projection as well as by the resulting introjection of good and bad objects. The ego, supported by the internalised good object and strengthened by the identification with it, projects a portion of the death instinct into that part of itself which it has split off – a part which thus comes to be in opposition to the rest of the ego and forms the basis of the super-ego.
>
> (p. 85)

Like Freud, Klein (1958) understood that an especially harsh superego was an obstacle to development and recovery. In her therapy with very young children she found a harsh superego present at an earlier age than Freud anticipated. Her child patients in their play revealed much more punitive internal parents in their minds than their actual parents whom she came to know. She saw it was the child's own aggressive feelings projectively attributed to the parents which could contribute to the introjection of a cruel superego. She noted how such a superego could crush the child's ego.

There continue to be differences between schools of psychoanalysis about the origins and development of the superego (Barnett, 2007), but wide agreement about the destructiveness of the superego, particularly in depression confirmed by psychoanalytic studies (Rosenfeld, 1959). Klein's followers pursued the study of destructiveness in the superego. Initially, Bion (1957), from his work with psychotic patients, described the destructiveness of the ego, but he later formulated an 'ego-destructive superego' Bion (1959) which develops as a result of problems in containment in early life. An absence of a containing mother or primary carer can be experienced as a cruel presence. If, instead of the infant's distress being transformed by mother's love and care, the distress remains unmodified, then what is internalised is a cruel parental object which strips away meaning and leaves the infant with a 'nameless dread'. Such problems in containment may arise because of mother's difficulties including envy and, or the infant's or child's envy. Rosenfeld (1987) confirmed Bion's views, describing an 'envious destructive superego' hidden in narcissistic omnipotent structures in the mind, which developed omnipotent phantasies in infancy to try to overcome helplessness when there were problems in holding and containment. Rosenfeld came to see that a destructive superego could be like a close-knit mafia gang. Rosenfeld described how the destructive superego can be disguised as benign and helpful; but its adverse character can become apparent when during the course of therapy it attempts to undermine any progress. O'Shaughnessy (1999) wrote of an 'abnormal' superego which is ruthless, takes the moral high ground but lacks morality.

Britton's (2003, 2020) further developments in understanding the destructiveness of the superego have been particularly influential to my approach. Britton describes the destructive superego as an 'internal saboteur' masquerading as a conscience 'claiming moral authority, proclaiming moral imperatives and dealing out punishments' (2020, p. 63). He discusses how some of the findings of neuroscience and models of the brain are consistent with the concept of an internal saboteur which is anti-life and in opposition to the self. Britton returns to Bion's insight about the way in which destructiveness gains the upper hand through its relationship with the ego. Bion saw the ego-destructive superego usurping the role of the ego. He understood the ego as the true moral arbiter, judge and observer, mediating between the internal and external worlds. Importantly Britton elaborates the therapeutic implications of this insight in the following way:

> The separation of the ego from the superego can only be achieved by the ego using its most valuable function – that of observation and

judgement – which it must turn on the superego… We must not simply
be judged by our conscience; we must subject conscience to judgement.

(2003, p. 101)

Commenting on the successful outcome of the analysis of one of his patients,
Britton concluded:

The emancipation of his ego from the adverse judgement of a potentially
envious superego was only achieved by the reclamation of his right to
form a judgement on his own internal critic. Even though this function
could not be silenced, it could be assessed.

(2003, p. 116)

Hence, an important element in my approach is to enable the ego to recognise, confront and free itself from the control of the destructive superego.
Instead of feeling the victim of persecutory guilt from a destructive
superego, the ego needs support to take responsibility and bear a depressive guilt for its own actions, which brings remorse and a wish to make
reparation.

Therapeutic Technique in My Approach

I aim in therapy to enable the patient to retrieve parts of the self lost in phantasy through projective identification, often because of persecutory guilt from
a destructive superego. Monitoring my counter-transference and studying the
clinical material can inform me about feelings which may be disowned, and
also inform me about the nature of the superego. The projection may not only
evoke the corresponding feelings in me but the projection may also include
the patient's disapproving superego that arouses my correspondingly disapproving superego in such a way that I also feel guilty about experiencing such
feelings and wish to disown them. I may need to struggle with feelings about
which my evoked superego makes me feel guilty. If I can remain curious and
observe my mind, I will then be in a position to begin to disentangle myself
from the projective processes between myself and my patient. Reflecting on
the nature of the feelings which may be evoked in me, including guilt from
my superego, can inform me about possible unconscious communication from
the patient. In the struggle with my superego I need to think about the kind of
guilt I experience whether a persecutory guilt from a destructive superego or
a depressive guilt in which my ego takes responsibility. I anticipate there will
be recurring struggles with my feelings, including guilt about the feelings,
as different aspects of myself may be evoked about similar struggles in my
patients. These struggles are externalised by the patient and experienced in
the transference and counter-transference relationship. During these times
I need to be able to bear the patient's projections and what may be stirred

within me as best I can, using self-reflection and supervision. I need to remain aware of my limitations and seek help when the need arises.

What is most often disowned are hateful, aggressive and other destructive aspects of ourselves which may derive from experiences of trauma, especially in early life and, or from innate factors. The disowning means that destructiveness may in phantasy be attributed to others who at times will include myself, and at times be enacted in reality when such feelings are actually evoked in me. Throughout life destructive external objects, whether the product of projections or reflecting their real nature, are often introjected as internal objects and form part of a destructive superego. I see a key therapeutic task as supporting the patient's ego in disentangling itself from the superego, and being able to observe and judge the superego, as well as itself. For this purpose, when interpreting, I think it useful to refer to the ego or self as 'you' and to find different ways of referring to what can essentially be an anti-life saboteur in the mind masquerading as a conscience.

The retrieving of projections takes place in the here-and-now of the transference relationship, as well as in then-and-there of extra-transference relationships in the patient's life. In so far as projections of destructiveness are withdrawn from others who are figures in the superego, the withdrawal of projections will diminish the superego's influence, the ego will be stronger and more able to take up its rightful place as judge and observer. This involves the painful work of mourning because it means acknowledging that destructiveness in oneself or others cannot be eliminated; the ego or self has to take responsibility for its own destructiveness, which may painfully bring sorrow, remorse and the wish to make reparation; and withdrawing projections from the therapist and others means acknowledging one's separateness and essential aloneness. Mourning also includes relinquishing projections from others, including our therapists, in order to be who we are and no-one else.

Finally, I would like to mention the role of love which is a cornerstone of our profession, but which I think is insufficiently acknowledged. However, it can be seen in Klein's emphasis on how the patient's own love mitigates hatred:

> I have earlier pointed out the threat, both to the self and to the analyst, arising in the patient's mind if split-off parts are regained in the analysis. In dealing with this anxiety one should not underrate the loving impulses when they can be detected in the material. For it is these which in the end enable the patient to mitigate his hate and envy.

(1975, p. 226)

Brenman Pick, referring to our aim as therapists to provide reliable care, writes:

When we show the patient that he becomes sadistic when he feels neglected or that he identifies himself with the neglecting object and fails to take note of the needy infantile self, I think whether we know it or not, the interpretation will contain some projection of our own wish to protect the baby from the sadistic part. The maintenance of a careful setting is in some way a demonstration of this care.

(1985, p. 161)

The danger of acting out an eroticised transference and counter-transference love which has long been recognised (Freud, 1915) perhaps inhibits appreciating the love in the care we provide. As well as recognising destructiveness in our patients, I believe it important to recognise our own and the patients' loving care which they give themselves by engaging in therapy.

Summaries of Parts of the Book

Part I Depression

Chapter I The Destructive Superego and Depression

The nature of destructiveness of the superego in depression is elucidated in Freud's description of its sadism, and Klein's and her followers' view of its envious character. The therapeutic implications of Kleinian developments are then discussed in one of Britton's case studies of the emancipation of the ego from the tyranny of the envious superego. I describe my thoughts about the retrieval of projective processes which enabled this emancipation and the consequent strengthening of the patient's ego. A case study of my own illustrates a struggle in a counter-transference influenced by the superego, and the necessary disentangling of projective processes between myself and the patient. The chapter concludes with a discussion about the implications for therapeutic technique.

Part II Death

Chapter 2 Dependency, Loneliness and Death

A discussion of fears of dependency, loneliness and death revealed in my therapy with patients who were suffering in old age. Fears of dependency were often exacerbated by a harsh superego, which had enabled a vulnerable self to prematurely hold itself together because of failures in the early dependency relationship. The apprehension can be that in becoming dependent in old age there will again be failures when needing care, an apprehension which can revive catastrophic anxieties. These anxieties resonate with the unconscious experience of death, and are concretely portrayed in the extreme dependency of advanced dementia. I discuss the implications of this understanding for carers and the support which they need but too frequently don't receive.

Chapter 3 Fears of Death and Fears of Dying

Fears of death and dying are explored in the counter-transference from my experiences supervising therapists working with terminally ill patients. Reflecting on the projective processes helped to differentiate between unconscious fears of dying and unconscious fears of death. Fears of dying resonated with failures in the early dependency relationship. Those fears were often exacerbated by a harsh superego, which was sometimes enacted in the relationships between carers and their patients. Fears of death were related to unthinkable annihilation of the self and nothingness. By contrast, in fears of dying the self survives. I discuss implications of understanding these fears in relation to therapeutic technique and setting ending dates for therapy with those who are suffering from terminal illnesses.

Part III Psychosis

Chapter 4 Violence and Psychosis

Projective identification is discussed as it can be understood in violence and psychosis from my work on two locked wards with patients who suffered from psychosis and were vulnerable to being violent. Vignettes illustrate how projective identification in violence conveyed emotional experiences for which there was little internal capacity for containment, because of early problems in the care giving relationship. Instead, emotional experiences were enacted in physical assaults on another's body, as though some kind of containment could only be achieved by physically forcing the experiences into someone else's body. These problems were associated with an agro-claustrophobic complex in which violent enactments were used as an attempt to overcome fears of closeness and separateness because of an underlying dread of annihilation. Psychotic organisations in the mind could be seen to bind together parts of a fragile sense of self, and offer psychic retreats from a dread of unintegration and fragmentation or depressive pain.

Chapter 5 Grief and Psychosis – The First Year of Therapy with J

The first year of a four-year therapy with a man, J suffering from psychosis. J was referred to me whilst he was an in-patient in an acute psychiatric unit. He attended as an out-patient. As he began to settle into the therapy, some depressive feelings about his sense of damage were soon followed by dreams indicating threatening internal figures, or sometimes apparently friendly ones,

denying his need of therapy and discouraging him about it. My interpretations aimed to support his ego or sane self which was painfully aware of the
damage he suffered, and differentiate it from a psychotic part which denied
the psychosis. When his ego was supported against this internal opposition,
he brought shocking details about the bleakness of his life. He tentatively
ventured into a painful process of trying to sort out what might be still possible for him. He also revealed how his ego was tempted to join in a collusive
way with the psychotic part.

Chapter 6 Encounters with a Psychotic Superego – The Second Year of Therapy with J

During this year I became consumed with feelings of fear and helplessness.
My supervisor helped me reflect on the counter-transference, and see how
a psychic retreat of a psychotic organisation which offered J a retreat from
depressive pain, included an omnipotent psychotic superego. This superego
ruthlessly attacked the therapy, at times trying to persuade J that death would
be better than depending on me. Sometimes J was rendered into what he
described as a zombie like state, a frightening experience of how the psychotic
superego can attack the mind itself. The attacks often followed any positive
developments. Managing to contain J's ensuing fear and hopelessness led to
hope and some developments. Eventually I was able to find a way of engaging
J's interest and curiosity about a little J, who was emerging in the therapy and
who was thinking things he'd not thought before.

Chapter 7 Struggles to Contain Madness – The Third Year of Therapy with J

Following a Christmas break, at the start of the year J suffered a psychotic breakdown. There were three more breakdowns during the first six
months, all requiring short term hospitalisation during which the therapy
continued. Each of the breakdowns was precipitated by an interruption in the
therapy. Between each breakdown there was some recovery. Much of the time
I struggled to think, unable to contain projections of 'beta elements', which
Bion described numb and deaden the mind in psychosis. I became identified
with J's mindless states. When, with the help of my supervisor I was able
to recover a capacity to think, J also began to recover. He did not suffer any
further breakdowns in the latter half of the year. Supervision enabled me to
re-establish a maternal holding for J's infant self.

Chapter 8 Mourning Omnipotence – The Fourth Year of Therapy with J

In the first six months of the fourth year, J brought signs of how he was
benefiting from therapy, for example in his ventures into more social and

lively relationships. In the latter part of the year a change in my personal life meant I decided to leave the unit, and could give just three months' notice. This news was devastating to J. Six weeks before the ending he withdrew from the therapy but remained in contact by email. Afraid of him breaking down, I tried to influence him to return to the consulting room, drawn into the phantasies of projective identification as though I could control his mind. When I was able to relinquish some of these omnipotent phantasies, bear my helplessness and acknowledge J' freedom and separateness, he and I were able to begin to mourn. J was able to convey feelings of gratitude and sadness without breaking down.

Part IV Life

Chapter 9 War

A cinematic study of a relationship between two soldiers from opposing sides in a civil war in the film *No Man's Land* prompted thoughts about projection and war. The relationship between the soldiers occurs as a result of their unexpected encounter in the no man's land which separates the warring sides. Following a shared moment of sorrow about the destruction of the natural world around them, these soldiers projectively attribute their hatred and murderousness to each other. The projections are accompanied by condemnation from destructive superegos which take the moral high ground. The soldiers' projectively enmeshed relationship presents a mirror of the projective relationship between the warring sides. An attempt at mediation by United Nations representatives, which might have brought some accord between the two sides and enabled some disentangling of the projections, fails because of this third party's vested interests and disowning of its destructiveness.

Chapter 10 The Holocaust

The novel *Beware of Pity*, written by a celebrated Jewish writer on the eve of the second world war, prompted thoughts about envy of Jews. The novel was a prescient warning about the dangers of denial of envy. The story begins before the start of the first world war. It shows how a soldier's sentimental pity for a young Jewish woman destroys her and her father at the outbreak of that war. The soldier's pity conceals his envy, which is projectively attributed to internal and external superego figures who express hatred for Jews. This family's tragedy reveals envy of the Jews as an important motive in the persecutors and murderers in the Holocaust, and how denial of envy and hatred probably contributed to the silence and inaction of others who were aware of the persecution and slaughter.

Chapter 11 Entitlement

The novel *The Uncommon Reader* about Queen Elizabeth II being transformed by becoming an avid reader, inspired thoughts about entitlement. The Queen's transformation begins when she reflects on her sense of entitlement, which included a lack of concern for others and supported her collusion with corruption. She begins to mourn and make reparation. I see the novel commenting about how, when we are identified with an infantile narcissism and omnipotence, we can collude with a society replete with entitlement and corruption. Mourning means being able to face the truth about our destructiveness as well as our love, and make reparation.

Chapter 12 Sexual Identity

The book concludes with my reflections on the novel *Nora Webster* about important changes in the life of a young widow which develop from her struggles in mourning. She sheds negative aspects of her identity which resulted from identifying with her husband's misogynistic projections. She begins to inhabit a sexual identity and mind of her own. I see misogynistic projections as an example of hated aspects of an innate bisexuality in our identities, which are projectively attributed to others. The recipients of such projections, particularly women and gay men become objects of hatred and forms of adverse treatment, and often internalise these negative identifications as aspects of their sexual identity in the form of misogyny or internal homophobia.

Notes

1 The articles were published in Routledge journals *Psychodynamic Practice* and *Psychoanalytic Psychotherapy*.
2 The articles were published in the Routledge journal *Psychodynamic Practice*.
3 Following Sedlak (2019), where seeking permission to use clinical material was not possible or would have had a detrimental impact on former patients, I have protected their confidentiality by disguising all identifiable details but at the same time retaining only non-identifiable details relevant to the clinical theme. Where it has been possible and appropriate to obtain permission, I have done so.

References

Barnett, B. (2007). *You Ought To! Psychoanalytic Study of the Superego and Conscience.* London: Karnac.

Bion, W. R. (1957). Differentiation of the psychotic from the non-psychotic personalities. *International Journal of Psycho-Analysis, 38,* 266–75.

Bion, W.R. (1959). Attacks on linking. *International Journal of Psycho-Analysis, 40,* 308–15.

Bion, W.R. (1962). The psychoanalytic study of thinking. *International Journal of Psycho-Analysis, 46,* 306–10.

Brenman Pick, I. (1985). Working through in the countertransference. *International Journal of Psychoanalysis, 66,* 157–66.

Britton, R. (2003). *Sex, Death, and the Superego.* London: Karnac.

Britton, R. (2020). *Sex, Death, and the Superego: Updating Psychoanalytic Experience and Developments in Neuroscience.* London: Routledge.

Freud, S. (1915). Thoughts for the times on war and death. *The Standard Edition of the Complete Psychological works of Sigmund Freud, Volume XIV* (pp. 273–300). London: Hogarth Press.

Freud, S. (1923). The ego and the id. *The Standard Edition of the Complete Psychological Works of Sigmund Freud, Volume XIX* (pp. 1–66). London: Hogarth Press.

Green, J. (1947). *If I Were You.* Michigan: Harper

Heimann. P. (1950). On counter-transference. *International Journal of Psychoanalysis,* 31, 81–4.

Hinshelwood, R. (1994) *Clinical Klein.* London: Free Association Books.

Joseph, B. (1987). Projective identification: Some clinical aspects. In E. Spillius & E. O'Shaughnessy (Eds) (2012). *Projective Identification: The Fate of a Concept.* London: Routledge.

Klein, M. (1946). Notes on some schizoid mechanisms. *International Journal of Psychoanalysis,* 27, 99–110.

Klein, M. (1955). On identification. In *The Writings of Melanie Klein Volume III.* London: Hogarth.

Klein, M. (1958). On the development of mental functioning. *International Journal of Psychoanalysis,* 39, 84–90.

Klein, M. (1975). Envy and gratitude. In *The Writings of Melanie Klein Volume III,* London: Hogarth.

Lemma, A. (2014). *Minding the Body: The Body in Psychoanalysis and Beyond.* London: Routledge.

Money-Kyrle, R. (1956). Normal countertransference and some of its deviations. *International Journal of Psychoanalysis, 37,* 360.

O'Shaughnessy, E. (1999). Relating to the superego. *International Journal of Psychoanalysis, 80,* 86 –70.

Rosenfeld, H. (1959). An investigation into the psychoanalytic theory of depression. *International Journal of Psychoanalysis, 40,* 105–29.

Rosenfeld, H. (1987). *Impasse and Interpretation.* London: Tavistock.

Sedlak, V. (2019). *The Psychoanalyst's Superegos, Ego Ideals and Blind Spots: The Emotional Development of the Clinician.* London: Routledge.

Sodre, I. (2012). Who's who? Notes on pathological identifications. In E. Spillius & E. O'Shaughnessy (Eds) (2012). *Projective Identification: The Fate of a Concept.* London: Routledge.

Spillius, E. (2012). Developments by British Kleinian analysts. In E. Spillius &
   E. O'Shaughnessy (Eds) (2012). *Projective Identification: The Fate of a Concept.*
   London: Routledge.
Steyn, L. (2013). Tactics and empathy: Defences against projective identification.
   International Journal of Psychoanalysis, 94 (6), 1093–113

Part I

Depression

Chapter 1

The Destructive Superego and Depression

Introduction

The following clinical vignettes illustrate aspects of the character of the destructive superego in depression:

A patient whom I saw for an assessment, who was suffering from depression and obsessional symptoms, complained of recurring nightmares. He recalled little about the nightmares but spoke of a scene from George Orwell's dystopian novel *Nineteen Eighty-Four* (1949) in which a man is held captive with a wire cage around his head. The cage has a funnel attached and a rat is crawling along the funnel towards the man's face. This image of torture by an omnipresent, totalitarian and persecuting regime vividly portrays the cruelty of his superego and its hold over the mind.

A trainee therapist whom I supervised told me about accompanying an elderly patient to the consulting room. Although physically fit his patient walked slowly and reluctantly. He began to feel uncomfortable because he found himself thinking he was leading a lamb to slaughter. His patient suffered from depression, had made several suicide attempts, previously dropped out of therapy and would do so again after a few sessions with the trainee. His counter-transference reveals how the patient's projections tuned into his frustration or hostility about her. His superego was evoked, condemned his feelings and made him feel guilty, as though he was about to murder an innocent patient; whereas a murderous superego in the client most likely contributed to her several suicide attempts, and killed off her ventures into therapy including the latest opportunity for therapy with the trainee (Terry, 2008).

In Freud's classic study of depression in 'Mourning and Melancholia' (1917) he observes how his depressed patients suffered from an 'extraordinary diminution' in self-regard and were consumed with self-reproaches. Freud understood these self-reproaches, which were often declaimed so publicly, were not about the self but unconsciously were accusations against a loved one whom the patient had lost. Part of the ego becomes identified with the lost loved one, 'the shadow of the (lost) object falls upon the ego' (p. 247). Freud described a

DOI: 10.4324/9781003319719-3

further splitting in the ego in which 'part of the ego sets itself over against the other, judges it critically'. Of this 'critical agency' he wrote:

'What we are here becoming acquainted with is the agency commonly called 'conscience'; we shall count it, along with the censorship of consciousness and reality-testing, among the major institutions of the ego, and we shall come upon evidence to show that it can become diseased on its own account.... In the clinical picture of melancholia, dissatisfaction with the ego on moral grounds is the most outstanding feature' (p. 247).

Freud's formulation of depression can be seen as a projective process in which a depressed client is unable to mourn because the loss is denied through an acquisitive form of projective identification with the lost loved one. In other words 'I haven't lost the loved one, I am the loved one'. The pain of the loss is also defended against by the superego's 'moral dissatisfaction' which is displaced onto the part of the ego identified with the lost loved one.

Klein's emphasis on the envious character of the destructive superego has been acknowledged particularly in relation to depression by Peter Fonagy, a psychoanalyst who plays a major role in research into psychotherapy. Fonagy (2008) celebrated Klein's contributions quoting her description of the envious superego:

'The super-ego figure on which strong envy has been projected becomes particularly persecutory and interferes with thought processes and with every productive activity, ultimately with creativeness' (Klein, 1957).

Fonagy describes how this insight helps reconcile a psychoanalytic phenomenological understanding of depression with the now well established view that there is a 'constitutional predisposition to depression'.

The relationship between the ego and the superego

Following Britton's development of Freud's concept of the ego, I use 'ego' to refer to the seat of integration between the self as experienced and the self as observed: 'the subjective self' integrated with the 'objective self'. Britton sees this integration as a result of the ego's capacity to take up a third position in triangular mental space, 'to observe oneself whilst being oneself' (2003, p. 91). Part of the ego is conscious and part unconscious. Britton writes that the worst outcomes occur when the ego identifies with a murderous superego, resulting in 'conscienceless killers' (2003, p. 120). Britton provides examples of his own work with patients who suffer from, but who are not identified with, murderous superegos. He also describes problems from less destructive superegos which reflect partial problems in early containment, and which result in an 'obstructing force in the mind that is felt to impede the way to understanding', and can underlie feeling 'blocked or stupid'(2003, p. 79). Britton gives an example of a benign superego in our professional lives as 'the trust of 'respected colleagues ... a source of inner strength', and indicates 'how very much we need good figures to have a place in that powerful internal moral position' (2003, p. 128).

The destructive superego is troubling not only because of its cruelty but also because it usurps the ego. As a consequence the ego needs to reclaim its proper function of self observation and judgement from the superego. Britton sees some biblical texts about God as studies of the superego, and cites the story of Job as a preoccupation with the place of evil in a world allegedly created by an omnipotent, benign God. Using post-modern translations of the original text, Britton gives a detailed analysis of Job to illustrate how the ego may achieve freedom from the dominance of the superego (2003, pp. 107–112). In the story Job's faith is sorely tested by being assailed with relentless personal losses, tragedies and afflictions. A turning point occurs when Job dares to make a judgement about God who could treat him in this way. This judgement unleashes God's fury that Job could so presume as to judge Him. Traditionally the story has been translated to suggest that Job repents in response to God's demonstration of His power and fury. Britton quotes contemporary translators who indicate a more correct translation is that Job gives an ironical response not a submissive one. This translation supports Britton's interpretation that Job, representing the ego, frees itself from domination by God, the superego. Britton sees this story 'represents a crucial moment in development when the ego takes the superego to task and, while still afraid of its power, claims the right to question its judgement and to doubt its motives' (2003, p. 111). From the perspective of projective processes is that Job's capacity to make a judgement of God illustrates how the ego has retrieved projections of its capacity for judgement and observation which were attributed to the superego.

Clinical illustrations of the emancipation of the ego from the dominance of a destructive superego

1. Mrs D – a case study from Britton

Britton uses this case study to demonstrate the emancipation of the ego from an envious superego (2003, pp. 121–125). I shall summarise the case study and comment from my view of the projective processes in the transference between patient and therapist, and between the patient's ego and superego, and the retrieval of projective identifications which are central to the ego achieving freedom from the tyranny of an envious superego.

Britton describes his patient, Mrs D as a professional academic who was suffering from depression. She was unable to fulfil her considerable potential particularly because of a writing block. Britton remarked on her truthfulness and strong loving feelings, qualities he mentions Klein singled out as especially helpful in mitigating envy. Britton outlines three phases which were repeated in cycles over a long analysis which was often beset by negative therapeutic reactions. He describes the first phase in terms of 'aspiration and inferiority', when he was experienced by Mrs D as capable of 'effortless superiority'. Britton was impressed by her endurance but appreciated she was judged internally as a 'failure' because of the effort required. In this phase Mrs D is projectively attributing a version of her own persecuting superego to Britton. Accordingly Britton was experienced as a superior God-like figure who need make no effort, judged her inferior because she needed to make effort, and who thereby stirred her envy. Such a superior analyst's expectations would be hard, if not impossible to achieve, and would inevitably be persecuting and only endorse her sense of failure. As a result of her envy, Mrs D projectively attributed to Britton a superiority which sought to maintain inferiority and envy in her.

In the second phase there was 'a mitigation of self-deprecation and an enhanced ability to work' which came with 'painful awareness of her envy'. Britton describes a sequence that became clear in which Mrs D would be in touch with her admiration for something he said, then would experience her hatred of him and wish that he would suffer in some way. She then felt remorseful. The working through that followed led to 'painful progress in her work and in the analysis'. In this phase Mrs D's ego is in touch with her admiration and hatred of what is good about Britton, and the ego retrieves and owns her projected envy. Her ego is thus less depleted, thereby stronger, able to take responsibility for envious attacks, experience guilt and remorse which leads to some reparation and restoration of her creative capacities. This retrieval of the projections externally from Britton and internally from her superego means that she is then more separate and more in touch with her own capacities.

Britton describes the third phase as a 'negative therapeutic reaction' which followed when Mrs D made progress, and was manifest in attacks on the therapy and especially on herself. Britton describes the attacks as beginning with a psychosomatic reaction which was associated with feelings she and Britton had failed, then a hypochondriacal reaction in which she became convinced she was suffering from a deadly illness. Britton gives an example of an occasion in which she was managing to write fluently and then believed she had some form of cancer. As they worked on these internal threats, she became aware of her wish to die, which was linked to her feelings of envy and disappointment about her own and others' capacities. Her suicidal feelings increased but she did not act on them out of concern not to 'inflict' that on Britton. During this phase there was much sorting through of her memories about her mother. Mrs D recalled her mother seemed to have been quite disturbed, at times cruel and envious of her as she reached adolescence. In this phase the attacks Mrs D makes on Britton and herself as a failed therapeutic couple come from an envious superego strengthened by envy reprojected from the ego into the superego. When her ego can again retrieve projected envy, despite fuelling death wishes, her ego is again stronger; she feels more separate, aware of and concerned for others. So, although she feels suicidal, she is able to resist the murderous impulses out of concern for Britton. This move into a depressive position is linked with her ego being less merged with and dominated by a murderous superego, and able to make more realistic appraisals of herself and her mother. These internal developments free her in the external world from the negative influence of her mother, as Britton wrote:

'The gradual displacement of the hostile internal object from its position as moral arbiter and the diminution of her actual mother's power to demoralise her moved in parallel' (2003, p. 125).

2. Mrs A – A case study from my practice

The context of this work was a specialist mental health service for people over the age of sixty-five in a unit including in-patient wards, a day hospital and out-patient services. In the interest of trying to respond to the diverse needs of patients, I explored longer gaps between sessions than the more usual practice of once weekly therapy. This flexibility also enabled me to reduce the waiting time for patients to be taken on for therapy. For a few patients who were unwilling to make a commitment to weekly sessions, when I suggested they chose the timing of the next session; some attended at monthly or longer intervals over a period of several years. This choice seemed to enable them to feel sufficiently held in a way they could manage and found helpful. Other patients like Mrs A found short term fortnightly sessions beneficial. The fortnightly sessions usually included a maximum of sixteen sessions which, with holiday breaks, covered a period of six to eight months. (For an extended discussion about this fortnightly model please see Terry, 2014.)

Mrs A was a white woman in her late seventies who was referred to me by her consultant psychiatrist to see if therapy could be useful for her. Mrs A had a life long history of bouts of depression. Previously, in mid-life she had some therapy which she found helpful. Her psychiatrist was worried Mrs A was slipping into another episode of depression. In the following case study of short term therapy with Mrs A I shall summarise and reflect upon the initial assessment meeting and each of the fifteen fortnightly sessions of the therapy, and include reflections on my counter-transference.

At the assessment meeting Mrs A described an unhappy life. She felt rejected by her mother and older brother. She felt close to her father but he was often absent because of his work. She married a man whom she found silent and withdrawn. He died early in the marriage leaving her with two young children. Mrs A continued working part-time in her chosen career until only a short time before I saw her. She suffered a great deal of pain from arthritis, and had concerns about increasing difficulties with her vision. She brought a dream which I interpreted as about her retirement and the loss of her work. Somewhat contemptuously she said 'Oh, it's all about retirement is it!' During this meeting I found myself feeling I did not like her and did not want to take her on for therapy. But I felt it was unreasonable to refuse to work with her, and there was no-one else to whom I could refer her. I offered to see her once each fortnight for short-term therapy. At the first therapy session a fortnight later, Mrs A said she was surprised I offered to see her because she thought I was angry with her. I did not confirm or deny this observation which I found uncomfortably perspicacious. She then spoke about her career, describing her good professionalism in a way I felt was drawing a contrast with my poor performance.

At the second session Mrs A immediately berated me for keeping her waiting and for being so silent. With exasperation she said she'd been surrounded by silence since she was a child. Other criticisms followed. I felt dismayed. According to my watch I was on time, and I thought I had been pretty active. Later in the session I said I thought Mrs A felt she couldn't depend on me, that she had to be self-sufficient and hold herself together. Mrs A was visibly moved by this interpretation and asked me why, as she thought over her life, she kept blaming herself. She gave examples and said her daughter tells her that the kind of things she blames herself for don't matter. I said I agreed with her daughter. At the end of the session, with a sense of despair, she said 'I am my own worst enemy'.

I was troubled about my dislike of Mrs A. Reflecting on the assessment meeting and the first session, I came to see Mrs A had projectively evoked a severe critic in me resulting in a hostile counter-transference. If, as a result of this counter-transference, I had referred her to another therapist I would have enacted that critical superego's denigration of her. When I could be curious about my reaction, I became capable of being more reflective about my feelings towards Mrs A. Importantly, as Caper (1999) has pointed out, at first I had to struggle with my own superego which was so critical. Mrs A's experience of observing me, consciously and unconsciously, struggling with my superego may have brought some hope that if I could manage to disentangle myself from my superego, then perhaps she could.

In the second session in relation to Mrs A's complaints about my keeping her waiting, I simply thought about the differences in our clocks. It did not occur to me I had kept her waiting for a fortnight in contrast to her previous experience of therapy which was probably weekly. I think such a thought was difficult for me to entertain because of a discomfort that however much I might try to justify the rationale for the fortnightly arrangement, it had aspects of an enactment of my feelings about not wanting to see her by spacing out the sessions. Later, my interpretation that she felt she had to hold herself together, brought a moment of closeness when she seemed to feel understood. Mrs A's subsequent question about why she kept blaming herself, was a significant shift from her blaming me about the time and so on. Perhaps her question was also an unconscious query about how I managed to free myself from a critical superego. She was clearly touched by my understanding of how hard it was to depend on me. In the interpretation I simply tried to describe my understanding of her experience of being with me. I tried not to deny her feeling that I could not be depended upon, which had some truth when I was feeling so critical of her. Caper (1999) describes this kind of interpretation as a 'holding' interpretation and Steiner (1993) an 'analyst-centred' interpretation, which mean describing the patient's experience of the therapist as a result of what the patient has projected, and at times evoked in the therapist.

At the third session Mrs A came saying she was feeling better. She said perhaps she was feeling better because of a change in medication; but later she said that when she found she was blaming herself in various ways she recalled I'd said those things didn't matter. I replied I agreed with her daughter. Then Mrs A went on to say 'As you said last time I am my own worst enemy'. I said I didn't think she was her own worst enemy, but I thought a part of her mind was her worst enemy. She was much surprised by this and several times asked me to explain what I meant. She brought a dream in which she was with her mother and brother. She was telling them off. (In the assessment meeting she described an unhappy childhood because of her mother and brother.) She walked away from them and was on a journey. She made her way to a railway station to buy tickets but discovered she had lost her handbag. Everyone was speaking in a language she couldn't understand. The ticket sellers were passive and did nothing to help her. I said it sounded like she was beginning to stand up to the worst enemy in her mind, which was represented by her mother and brother in the dream. I said it seemed I was like the ticket sellers who were so passive and unhelpful. She laughed heartily in agreement.

In this first part of this third session Mrs A confirmed, somewhat ambivalently, some benefit from the previous session, which I see resulted from my supporting her ego to stand up against blame from her superego. She then recalled I said she was her own worst enemy. Following my clarification that I did not think of her like that but differentiated between a worst enemy in her mind and herself, she brought a dream which confirmed her standing up to her worst enemy superego. Her depiction of me in the dream as a passive, unhelpful ticket seller unconsciously confirms my earlier, therapist-centred interpretation of how I was a therapist on whom she could not depend. This denigratory view of me had persisted despite her experience of feeling some benefit from the therapy, and suggests an envious quality in her superego trying to spoil the good she had felt from the therapy. Her laughter in agreement to my interpretation of the denigration signalled some insight, in the way humour often reflects a capacity to step back and observe oneself or others, and be amused at our follies and tragedies. In this way Mrs A revealed her capacity for insight. Steyn (2016) describes patients like Mrs A as less disturbed because they are able to recognise projections when interpreted. By contrast Steyn describes more disturbed patients who use a 'more total form' of projective identification to rid themselves entirely of what is projected with the result that the projection feels 'foreign' (p. 1097). Steyn sees less disturbed patients maintaining an 'as if' nature of the transference, which is lost for more disturbed patients who remain convinced of the reality of their projected experience.

At the latter part of the third session Mrs A brought a dream which reminded her of the loneliness she felt throughout her life. She had few friends. She was lonely as a child and recalled a photo of herself on her own. Then she remembered she was smiling in the photo. She said her father had taken the photo. (In the assessment she told me she felt close to her father but said he was often at work away from home.) I said she wasn't on her own because she was with her father. I talked about how the dreams revealed negative propaganda spread by this worst enemy in her mind, suggesting I was passive and useless to her and she might as well be on her own; whereas she had the thought the sessions with me were helpful to her, perhaps she was even enjoying them.

In the latter part of the third session Mrs A's associations show her pursuing the implications of her insight about the transference distortions in the dream. She was able to disentangle some of the distortions in the narrative of her past, she was not always miserable and alone and, in the transference, in the here-and-now I help her like her father when I show her pictures of herself with me. The interpretations supported her ego to assert realistic observations freed of the superego's spoiling propaganda.

At the fourth session Mrs A spoke again about her loneliness. She went to a meeting of a group for older women. She described the women in a way I found amusing and laughed with her. I became uncomfortable because I realised I was joining in mocking the women. I said I felt she was ridiculing the women and was reminded of Groucho Marx who said any club that would have him as a member he wouldn't want to join. She laughed. At the next, fifth session she came back saying she'd been thinking about what I said about ridiculing the women and Groucho Marx. She said she recognised these things in herself and did not like them. During this session I reminded her we were now nearly half way through the therapy and confirmed the ending date.

In the fourth session, encouraged by Mrs A's reflectiveness I risked an explicit interpretation of her envious denigration. This is an example of what Caper (1999) describes as a 'containing' interpretation which can be made when the patient can manage recognising the therapist's separateness and freedom to have a different view. Steiner (1993) describes these interpretations as 'patient-centred interpretations' when the therapist can make interpretations which help the patient understand their contribution to their difficulties and when they are therefore able to retrieve projections. I approached the interpretation in an indirect way by interpreting her transference relationship to the older women in the group, sometimes described as an 'extra-transference' interpretation'. Extra-transference interpretations are frowned upon in some psychoanalytic circles, but in his seminal paper on effective interpretations

Strachey (1934) acknowledged the usefulness of extra-transference interpretations. Intuitively I included some humour about Groucho Marx. With hindsight I think I was apprehensive about interpreting the envy in her mockery of the group, especially because she might hear the interpretation as a condemnation of her from my superego. The joke helped her step back and, in the laughter, observe herself like Groucho Marx. Mrs A showed how she held the sessions in mind and reflected on them between the sessions. She was able to mull over the interpretation and reach a painful recognition of her envy The ownership of her envy was a breakthrough because instead of internally feeling the victim of an envious superego, and externally of other people when her envy was projectively attributed to them, her ego was taking responsibility for its envy.

Much later, after the therapy with Mrs A was concluded I came to understand more about the source of my initial dislike of her. I recalled that in the first therapy session she said she was surprised I offered to see her for therapy. She thought I was angry with her when she asked me in the assessment session about the difference between a psychiatrist and a psychologist. When she gave this explanation, I realised I had forgotten her asking the question. I think the question very likely provoked difficult feelings in me about the differences between the two professions of psychology and psychiatry. I have a lower position in that pecking order. The question stirred uncomfortable feelings of envy. My discomfort reflected my own superego's disapproval of such feelings. Her question and my reaction were repressed, but I was left with a strong disapproval of Mrs A. Reflecting on how my superego was evoked in the countertransference freed me of its influence, and enabled me to engage constructively in the therapy with Mrs A to reach an understanding of how troubled she was by her superego. But I failed to understand the source of my disapproval because of the strength of my superego's condemnation of envy. I was thus prevented from recognising Mrs A's early unconscious communication specifically about her struggles with her envy and her superego's condemnation of it. Only with hindsight could I see she had projectively communicated about her envy and her superego's disapproval of it by evoking my envy and my superego's disapproval of it. My dislike of her was an enactment of my superego's condemnation of myself and my envy.

Steyn (2016) has written eloquently of our struggle as therapists to bear what patients find loathsome about themselves when this means trying to bear loathsome aspects of ourselves, which are evoked in the counter-transference through projective identification. In a searching case study of her own difficulties, Steyn describes defences against projective identifications. For example when apparently making an analyst-centred interpretation a therapist might say 'You feel I am angry with you…' in such a way as to imply the patient is mistaken. The therapist may be denying the truth of the patient's experience because what has been evoked in the therapist felt unacceptable. As I have indicated, I believe an aspect of these difficulties is that what is included in the projected feelings is a superego condemnation of the feelings. The projection evokes condemnation from the therapist's superego about similar feelings in the counter-transference. So as therapists we can come to feel we shouldn't have those feelings. It can then be hard to maintain an attitude of curiosity about our feelings, and explore the possible communicative aspects of the counter-transference feelings including the sense of condemnation.

At the sixth session Mrs A brought a dream which was about her retirement. Discussing the dream she became sad. For the first time she acknowledged how much her work meant to her and how much she missed it. She then spoke of a relative who was 'jealous' of her success at work.

In this sixth session Mrs A's dream about retirement echoed the first dream she brought at the assessment session. In contrast to her difficulty in considering her feelings about retirement at that time, Mrs A was able to be in touch with her sadness about the loss of her work. The loss, signalled by the dreams, was probably linked to what her psychiatrist feared would be another episode of depression. Mrs A's denigration of herself and her achievements had its source in an envious superego. The denigration protected her from envy projected into others, as though there was little about her to be envied. When she was able to own her projected envy, she was able to realistically appraise her success and the value of her career. The withdrawal of the projections of envy into others meant, when such figures were re-introjected into her superego, the superego would be thereby weakened. Owning her envy made her ego was stronger and less vulnerable to being dominated by the superego. Consequently she was in a better position to maintain realistic appraisals of herself and others.

In recognising her relative's 'jealousy' Mrs A appreciated how enviable her work had been, and she was able to feel sadness about its loss. Her envious superego's relentless criticisms about her work protected her from the depressive pain of losing a career in which she had been successful and from which she derived much satisfaction. Mrs A's denigration of her work illustrates how the envious superego's denigration enabled her to try to overcome the pain of loss and mourning, but at the same time this meant she was then vulnerable to becoming depressed.

I assumed Mrs A's use of the word jealousy to describe her cousin's envy, reflected a popular usage, in which envy and jealousy are sometimes confused and used interchangeably. On reflection, perhaps Mrs A intuited how her cousin was jealous of Mrs A's love of her work as well as envious of the good work Mrs A had achieved, and wanted to spoil Mrs A's relationship with her work. Usually jealousy refers to a triangular relationship in which one person is aggrieved about the loss of the loved one to another. The joining of envy and jealousy can be seen to have spoiling, even murderous consequences when jealousy leads to murder of either or both the loved one and the other who has displaced the jealous person.

Mrs A's dream about the loss of her work in the sixth session was probably triggered in the transference by my reminder in the previous session about the ending date of therapy, we were then half way through. I didn't interpret the dream in terms of the transference relationship but stayed with the sad feelings which she was able to feel when she did not denigrate what or whom was lost. Her sadness indicated a depressive move into mourning instead of becoming depressed. There was much to mourn, the loss of her career, the ageing of her body, ultimately the loss of her own life, and in the here-and-now, the ending of the therapeutic relationship.

At the seventh session Mrs A described how she had been to a family wedding. It had been some time since she had seen the people who were present. She was shocked to see how much her relatives had aged. I interpreted the shock of recognising her own ageing, and that time was running out in her life and in the therapy. She spoke of difficulties getting on with anything or knowing just what she wants to do with the time that is remaining. In a rather wistful way, she wondered why she couldn't get on with things. I said, 'Well, we could spend time thinking about it, but perhaps that's the kind of rumination which has to be stopped so you can get on with things'. Later, I said perhaps if she really took seriously that time was running out, she might know what she wants to do in the time that is left. She replied that as she tries to think of what she wants to do her mind goes blank, she has no idea. Towards the end of the session, she said she found herself thinking of her longing to travel. I said, 'Well, what are you waiting for!' She laughed.

At the eighth session Mrs A spoke about her experience of raising her children, and her son's and daughter's families and successes. She said she'd noticed how much she is drawn back to thinking about the past, and is inclined to criticise herself for not doing better. I said that this takes her away from the present and enjoying what she has achieved. I confirmed the dates for the Christmas break which was in a month's time. At the ninth session, the penultimate one before the break, she was in a lighter, playful mood. She described feeling 'euphoric' because in her garden, which she loved, she'd noticed a robin who accompanied her when she was gardening. The robin kept an eye on her. Later, she talked about a minor traffic scrape which occurred when parking her car, and she added with a laugh, 'But I'm not beating myself up about it'. I said I thought she was managing the 'worst enemy' in a better way, not dominated by it. She agreed, but added 'not completely'. In the tenth and final session before the break, Mrs A talked of difficulty in asking her daughter for help, and later finding herself singing when the daughter was helping her with some clearing up. She spoke of her enduring arthritic pain and worries about her declining mobility. Towards the end of the session she talked of how unsupported she felt by her husband because he didn't talk to her.

Confirming the ending date and the imminence of a holiday break in these latter sessions galvanised Mrs A's thinking about making the most of the time left in the therapy and in her life. Quinodoz (2010) has written about how older people can get stuck in deadly grooves as a defence against recognising advancing time and the approach of the end of life, as though going round and round in circles can prolong life and avoid death. I felt encouraged by the story of the robin who accompanied Mrs A in her garden because I understood it as a reference to myself in the transference. I had become a helpful internal object with whom she was becoming identified in observing her mind, especially how her envious superego can attack her. In the last session before the holiday, the anticipation of my abandonment of her stirred denigration of me. In the transference I was felt to be like her silent husband whom she lost early in her married life. She was again vulnerable to an envious superego's denigration to try to alleviate the pain of loss.

After the Christmas break Mrs A was unable to resume therapy on the eleventh session because of heavy snowfalls. This meant it was six weeks before I saw her again at the twelfth session. She said Christmas had been difficult, but unlike previous Christmases she didn't get depressed. She noticed she was drawn to critically going over the past, but often succeeded in stopping herself doing so and was able to get on with other things. She made plans to visit an art gallery with a friend and to have a short holiday abroad with her daughter.

In this twelfth session I was encouraged to hear Mrs A had not become depressed. It was evident she was maintaining an identification with an observing ego, noticing herself being attacked by the superego, and thereby better able to withstand the attacks which otherwise could have led to depression.

At the thirteenth session, which was the third last session, Mrs A came saying she still had problems about 'no motivation'. She talked in a despairing way about the problems of ageing, particularly her struggle with arthritis and mobility. She described wishing she would simply not wake up in the morning. She found herself thinking there was no point in continuing her daily exercises even though she knew she felt better after she did them. I said it seemed to me it wasn't so much an absence of something called motivation, but more the presence of a destructive force in her mind which undermines her and tries to persuade her she'd be better off dead.

In this thirteenth session as we neared the ending of the therapy, there was a regressive return to the beginning, as though nothing had been achieved, which Freud (1937) recognised as a plea not to end the therapy. For Mrs A this included a resurgence of an envious superego which tried to promote despair and erase any hope. She was not actively suicidal. Her passive death wishes were aspects of internal envious attacks.

At the fourteenth, penultimate session, she talked of better contact with her daughter who had again been helping her clear things out, and who surprised her by giving her a big hug. She brought a dream in which she was in a large house which was like the building in which she had worked. She was sorting and clearing things out. She said there were many rooms, some of which she could no longer enter, and she felt she was too old and there were things she could no longer do.

In this fourteenth session, there was some recovery as she felt supported by her daughter in the clearing out work and by myself in the transference. The dream confirmed the clearing out work continuing in her mind, and that she was more able to face what was and was not possible for her at that stage of her life and the therapy. She was not depressed but was mourning the end of her career, her life and the therapy.

At the fifteenth, final session, Mrs A brought some flowers. She said they were not the flowers she had hoped to bring. The poor weather prevented her from going out to get the ones she had in mind, which she specially liked because they were 'simply themselves, no frills or decorations'. She brought a dream in which a young girl was lying in a rowing boat out at sea, and thinking with resignation that she was dying. She looked up and saw a huge liner which had come to rescue her. Mrs A then talked of how much she'd appreciated and benefitted from the therapy. She had recently joined a large organisation linked with her religion which would give her access to a range of clubs and activities. She spoke of feeling there was more she could pursue. She mentioned her interest in reading reviews of books she has read. She was often struck by the reviewers' insights and returned to the texts to think about those insights. She looked forward to having the opportunity, through the clubs, of being able to discuss such things with others.

Concluding reflections about therapeutic technique

When as therapists we are recipients of projections of a destructive superego, a particular difficulty we face is that these projections can evoke our own superego in the counter-transference. Caper (1999) gives various illustrations of how, when evoked, the therapist's superego can interfere with making an effective interpretation because the therapist becomes concerned about losing a 'good' relationship with the patient, or about not being 'tactful' or 'empathic'. Citing Strachey's (1934) seminal work on the difficulties of making a mutative interpretation, Caper describes how the therapist may sometimes resort to giving advice or reassurance, and may undermine an interpretation by making two interpretations at the same time, or by giving an interpretation in an attitude expressing scepticism about its content. The therapist may be inclined in interpretations to take the side of the patient against others such as their parents and judge the parents harshly. Caper understands these kind of problems as a result of the therapist's intimidation and fearfulness of the patient's destructive superego, which takes the moral high ground, lacks morality and is not interested in reality.

Caper is clear that what the patient needs is the therapist's ego to simply state the truth as the therapist sees it. In order to achieve this capacity therapists have to disentangle their own ego from their superego. Caper has developed much clarity about this internal disentangling which he understands we achieve by virtue of our relationship to psychoanalysis, meaning study, training, supervision and personal therapy. This relational link in the mind supports the therapists' receptiveness to the patient's projective identifications, and enables therapists to disentangle themselves from projective identifications. The therapeutic disentangling is especially hard because of the nature of the projective identification. The unconscious phantasy of invasion and control in projective identification enslaves the ego to the superego, which means the destructive superego can possess the mind. In order to relinquish phantasies of possession and control, therapist and patient need to be able to mourn omnipotence and separateness. Withdrawing projections aimed at possession and control means recognising the freedom of loved and hated objects in the internal and external worlds, a freedom to be surprised and amazed at one's mind (Caper, 1997).

My case study of Mrs A included examples of technique Caper (1999) and Steiner (1993) have elaborated which are especially relevant to therapy when there is a destructive superego. They propose ways of formulating inter-pretations according to how much the patient's mind is in the grip of the superego. Particularly, but not only in the early stages of therapy, they rec-ommend aiming to give the patient the experience of being understood, by offering holding (Caper) or therapist-centred (Steiner) interpretations which merely describe the patient's experience of the therapist. These interpret-ations can be seen as modelling the ego's capacity to observe oneself whilst being oneself, and of demonstrating the therapist is able to bear the patient's projections without precipitously trying to enable the patient to retrieve projections.

Following developments in the therapy, particularly when the patient can bear the reminder of separateness when offered a different point of view, and step back to observe the mind, then it is possible to venture patient-centred' (Steiner) or 'containing' (Caper) interpretations. In this kind of interpretation the therapist offers observations of the patient's feelings and behaviour in rela-tion to the therapist or others, in order to promote the patient's capacity to understand. If such interpretations are made when the patient is projectively merged with the therapist and attributes their destructive superego to the therapist, on the one hand these interpretations are likely to be experienced and probably rejected as moralistic condemnations from the therapist's superego. On the other hand the patient may be inclined to reframe the inter-pretation as a confirmation of their own view, and reassurance of a merger with the therapist in which there are no differences or separateness. Such a perfect unity of understanding can carry an implication that understanding brings forgiveness as though, as Caper says 'to understand everything is to forgive everything'. This state of mind which denies separateness, may be a merger with an idealised superego in the therapist which can bestow forgiveness. Such a state of mind may find matching projections in a therapist who seeks to encourage an idealised transference particularly when intimidated by a patient's persecuting superego. The shadow of this destructive superego's moralistic condemnations of the self and others needs to be explored, to sort truth from lies and what may or may not bring remorse and sorrow and the wish to make reparation.

Caper (1999) sees working through in therapy involves painful awareness that destructiveness in oneself cannot be deleted. Britton (2003) understands that emancipating the ego from a destructive superego does not mean destructiveness is vanquished. To paraphrase Britton, the terrorists are still present but at least they're not running the show. Caper notes it is the destructive superego which drives projective identification. Effective interpretations strengthen the ego by enabling the retrieval of projected capacities. The patient is thereby strengthened to take responsibility for hatred and destructiveness, to take pride in love, creativity and achievements, and to accept that one is only who one is and no-one else. In Klein's lectures on technique she pointed out that love which can acknowledge hatred is much richer than love which denies it (Steiner, 2017).

References

Britton, R. (2003). *Sex, Death, and the Superego.* London: Karnac.

Caper, R. (1999). *A Mind of One's Own.* London: Routledge.

Fonagy, P. (2008). Being envious of envy and gratitude. In P. Roth & A. Lemma (Eds) *Envy and Gratitude Revisited* (pp. 201–10). London: Karnac.

Freud, S. (1917). Mourning and melancholia. *The Standard Edition of the Complete Psychological Works of Sigmund Freud, XIV* (pp. 237–58). London: Hogarth Press.

Freud, S. (1937). Analysis terminable and interminable. *The Standard Edition of the Complete Psychological Works of Sigmund Freud, XXII* (pp. 209–54). London: Hogarth Press.

Fonagy, P. (2008). Being envious of envy and gratitude. In P. Roth & A. Lemma (Eds) *Envy and Gratitude Revisited* (pp. 201–10). London: Karnac.

Klein, M. (1957) Envy and gratitude. In *The Writings of Melanie Klein Volume III.* London: Hogarth.

Orwell, G. (1949). *Nineteen Eighty Four.* London: Penguin.

Quinodoz, D. (2010). *Growing Old: A Journey of Self-discovery.* London: Routledge.

Steiner, J. (1993). *Psychic Retreats: Pathological Organisations of the Personality in Psychotic, Neurotic and Borderline Patients.* London: Routledge.

Steiner, J. (2017). *Lectures on Technique by Melanie Klein: Edited with Critical Review by John Steiner.* London: Routledge.

Steyn, L. (2013). Tactics and empathy: Defences against projective identification. *International Journal of Psychoanalysis, 94* (6), 1093–113.

Strachey, J. (1934). The nature of the therapeutic action of psycho-analysis. *International Journal of Psychoanalysis, 15*, 127–59.

Terry, P (2008). *Counselling and Psychotherapy with Older People: A Psychodynamic Approach*. London: Palgrave Macmillan.

Terry, P. (2014). Not too late: Fortnightly short term dynamic therapy with older people. *Psychodynamic Practice, 20* (4), 362–72.

Part II

Death

Chapter 2

Dependency, Loneliness and Death

Introduction

Working with people suffering from the physical and mental onslaughts of old age I saw three overlapping and interacting fears: dependency, loneliness and death. These fears are not exclusive to old people but are often linked with old age. Initially I worked with people described as the 'elderly physically or mentally frail' who were in a geriatric hospital. Some years later I worked in a specialist mental health service for 'older adults'. The various euphemisms used to describe old people are indicative of the frightening spectres they present about what threatens us all about old age, most especially our death. I prefer to simply refer to these people as old because undoubtedly their suffering was exacerbated by old age.

I saw the importance of thinking about and working with the carers of old people. Winnicott (1971, p. 587) famously once said 'There is no such thing as an infant' which he later explained meant 'that whenever one finds an infant one finds maternal care, and without maternal care there would be no infant'. Much the same can be said of someone suffering the effects of old age. The carer's role is often vital to the survival and well-being of the old person, except the strains of providing the care are usually greater because the old person faces increasing decline and ultimate death. Moreover, as I will illustrate, fears about dependency, loneliness and death are often projectively evoked in the carers who, without adequate support, are vulnerable to returning the projections.

Dependency

Peter Hildebrand (1995) pioneered therapy with elderly people at the Tavistock Clinic in London. Early in this work he made a video recording of his experience with an eighty-nine-year-old white woman. At first, he only agreed to see her for a few exploratory sessions because of his reservations about whether therapy would be feasible with someone of her advanced age. Watching the recording it was riveting to see this woman relishing being

DOI: 10.4324/9781003319719-5

listened to and thought about. She grasped Hildebrand's words with delight. Hildebrand was clearly also enjoying the experience. He continued to see her for weekly therapy sessions until she died two years later. Hildebrand's patient had led a formidable and healthy life. She was referred to Hildebrand after she suffered a severe physical illness. Although she recovered her physical health it was as though, psychologically, she collapsed. She was subsequently unable to resume her independent, active life. I was reminded of Hildebrand's patient when I started seeing old people and met a white woman, Mrs T who was remarkably active into her eighties (Terry, 2008). She continued to help in the family business, often lifting heavy machinery, at the same time as house-keeping and gardening for her family. She suffered an attack of shingles and, though making a good recovery, she withdrew to her flat and spent most of the day lying on a sofa, weak and breathless, apparently unable to do anything for herself.

My subsequent therapeutic experience with old patients confirmed a pattern in which people, who have often led exceptional lives, in old age can suddenly become psychologically debilitated by the onset of a physical illness or other intimations of dependency. Brian Martindale (1989) wrote a seminal article which illuminates the underlying dynamic. He describes the experience of becoming dependent again in old age as presenting par-ticular problems when there have been failures in the dependency relationship early in life. The approach of dependency, heralded by the decline in physical and mental capacities, brings fears that once again dependent needs will not be met. Martindale noted these fears can be projectively communicated to therapists and others who consciously or unconsciously can dread patients becoming dependent on them, which may also tune into worries the therapists may have about their own parents. These fears can lead to difficulties in old people receiving the help they need, for example by being referred from one professional to another. Old patients who collapsed into helplessness seem to have held themselves together and avoided depending on others until those ways of managing their fears were punctured by painful reminders of vulner-ability and dependency.

Psychoanalytic infant observation studies reveal how fears of dependency resonate with early problems of holding and containment. Esther Bick (1968) drew attention to the importance of the capacity of the mother or primary carer to hold the infant in mind, gather together the different fragments of the infant's experience and give them coherence, just as the skin holds together all the different parts of the infant's body. If there are problems in holding then the infant, child and later adult may develop premature ways of holding him or herself together, in order to try to manage a dread of 'unintegration'. Bick used the term unintegration to describe 'catastrophic anxieties in the uninte-grated state as compared with the more limited and specific persecutory and depressive ones' (1968, p .484). These anxieties are also discussed in relation to psychosis in Part III.

Mrs T would usually begin her sessions addressing me with a pleading look to help her unbutton her coat. Although there was some physical basis for Mrs T's debilitated state, her doctors were puzzled by how helpless she had become. Her family were disbelieving about her weakened state and complained she was malingering. I struggled with similar doubts when I prevaricated about whether to help her unbutton her coat, or when she would ask for a glass of water as though she were about to expire. I felt ashamed of having such doubts and not immediately offering to help this old woman. The counter-transference gives some indication of how Mrs T's superego took her to task about her dependency. This kind of superego, though ruthless, nonetheless had been a source of internal strength with which she had held herself together. It doubtless drove her to remarkable achievements, and helped her avoid depending on others lest once again she would be let down. When this superego was projectively evoked in others like myself or members of her family, it could lead to an enactment of those fears. Her dependency could be dismissed as malingering, as though no-one could bear to know about it, and understandably she felt let down again. I became very fond of Mrs T and enjoyed working with her. Sadly, Mrs T died several months after I started seeing her.

I was asked to talk to staff in a nursing home about one of their residents. Mrs C had become rude and aggressive to the staff, often shouting insults at them and fellow residents. When staff tried to discuss these problems with her, she insisted there was nothing the matter and that she would not talk to anyone else. She began refusing to walk, holding onto the sides of her wheelchair as though she was frightened she would fall out of it. She had an exceptional general knowledge and was keenly aware of everything happening in the nursing home. Recently a nurse, to whom she had become close, had left the nursing home. I learnt that as the eldest of a large family she had looked after her younger siblings. Later, she became a carer in nursing homes. I talked to the staff about all the losses in this woman's life, including the loss of her own home and independence, and most recently the nurse on whom she had depended. I said I thought she had probably held herself together from a young age and throughout her life, perhaps through her exceptional grasp of general knowledge and through caring for others. The recent loss of her nurse may have been the last straw, and revived infantile and other losses.

It seemed to help the staff bear Mrs C's abusive behaviour when they could see that her harsh words and aggressive behaviour could be a way of stiffening herself, and trying desperately to hold herself together again. When old people were cruel in their criticisms and attitudes. I found it useful to reflect on the helplessness and a dread of unintegration they were trying to manage, and how their attacks could be a means of survival (Symington, 1985). I saw these attacks as taking refuge in a strong and harsh superego as a way of holding themselves together. The image of Mrs C tightly holding onto the sides of a wheelchair, which she didn't need, vividly portrays the dread of unintegration, of being unheld and falling to pieces. Whilst appreciating the revival of an infantile dread in old people it was important not to infantilise them or overlook their long life experience.

Loneliness

Noel Hess (1987), writing about fears of loneliness for old people, draws attention not only to the fear of losing a partner, family and friends but also the 'terror' of being left alone 'without an organising and containing part of the self, which is felt to be lost in the catastrophes of old age: stroke, injury, illness and dementia' (p. 214). Hess discusses tyrannical behaviour that can result from such catastrophes and the ensuing fears of dependency and helplessness. He illustrates tyranny in Shakespeare's King Lear and clinical examples of patients referred to him by their general practitioners. Tyrannical behaviour is characterised by a need to control others and is reminiscent of Mrs C described earlier. I see tyrannical behaviour as the use of projective identification to rid the self of an unbearable helplessness, and to possess and control. When helplessness is projectively evoked in others then they can be controlled and made dependable, and this overcomes fears of dependency. In this way tyrannical behaviour is an example of what Klein described as a manic defence which can include control, contempt and triumph.

In a case study of loneliness Hess (2004) describes a woman in her sixties who suffered from depression. She was referred for therapy to a clinical psychologist. He was in his thirties, an experienced clinician but with relatively little experience of psychotherapy. She phoned him to confirm her appointment. From that first contact she made it clear she thought he was too young and inexperienced. Despite these reservations she agreed to see him. During the meeting her complaints continued, but the therapist managed to make some contact with her when he spoke about her loneliness. She then told him she was suffering from a degenerative disease which would only worsen as she aged. She said she would attend the next appointment because she was interested in what he had said about her loneliness. At that appointment she resumed her criticisms. She remonstrated about the therapist's surname saying he obviously belonged to a nationality who had persecuted members of her race. She did not attend again. She wrote to say she was unhappy about the age gap between them and had arranged to be referred to another therapist.

Hess' case illustrates how a destructive superego can exacerbate problems of loneliness and dependency, which can also be seen in Mrs A's experience of loneliness described in Chapter 1. This therapist was left in no doubt about the persecuting nature of his patient's superego which attacked him relentlessly. The patient's destructive superego was full of contempt for the therapist's vulnerabilities about being much younger and inexperienced. This gave him a painful experience of how his patient's vulnerabilities, whether for example her lack of friends or becoming helpless and dependent, were reviled in her mind. Although the therapist showed some understanding of her loneliness, he probably did not appreciate that in the grip of her superego she was likely to hear his interpretations as criticisms. Nor perhaps did he appreciate how the patient may have projectively evoked his own superego which may have given reality to a feeling of being criticised by him.

When an old person has suffered severe trauma and not been able to speak of it, there can be a terror of dying alone with all the trauma in one's mind. Mr K was a survivor of a concentration camp and had not previously spoken of his experience in the camp until he engaged in therapy with me. He brought an urgency to speak about his experience and a fear he would not be able to do so. He struggled for a considerable time to begin to talk about what had happened in the camp. When he finally began to do so I became ill, and at short notice had to cancel the next week's session. I soon recovered and was able to return the following week. I was worried he would not be able to resume, but he continued his story almost as though there had been no interruption. To an extent Mr K managed being in the camp by dissociating himself from what was happening, as though he was a bystander looking on in disbelief. He needed to tell his story to make it real, but feared I would be an onlooker too. I think my illness and absence was probably a relief because it was evidence of the impact and reality of the horrendous trauma he had suffered. Talking about his experiences was indeed hard for him and myself to bear, but doing so eventually was beneficial for him (Terry, 2008).

Death

Valerie Sinason (1992) has written a moving account of psychoanalytic therapy with a man whom she began seeing whilst he was in the early stages of dementia. Sinason pioneered psychoanalytic work with handicapped children and adults. She developed an important understanding of how organic impairment can be exacerbated by emotional factors, contributing to what she described as a 'secondary handicap'. She came to appreciate how 'a real organic loss shared a parallel existence with temporary emotionally caused impairment' (1992, p. 97). When she was able to recognise and interpret her patient's anger, he was able to remember words he had forgotten, and sometimes to resume speaking in coherent sentences. Quite early in the therapy he spoke about his fears for the future. He asked if life would have any meaning if someone didn't know they were alive. Sinason replied, 'That would indeed be a death, to be stripped of meaning. It would be a death of the mind' (p. 102). The patient nodded. He said 'Good' twice in reply to express his appreciation of her words. Sinason brought a receptiveness for his worst fears as he anticipated the dreadful losses suffered in advanced stages of dementia: extreme dependency, losing all independent capacities of language and bodily function, with perhaps little or no memory. These fears for which Sinason gave words about a death of the mind, doubtless accompany the news of a dementia diagnosis. There can be no reassurance against the feared outcome. Sinason shows reassurance can come from being with someone who can bear to take in, think about and articulate the feared worst, which may help the person suffering from dementia to bear what feels unbearable.

I shall describe an observation made of people in transition between suffering early and advanced stages of dementia who were patients in a residential dementia unit. They were in the dayroom. A relative was also present. The observation was made by a clinical psychology trainee who as part of her training visited the dementia unit each week and brought her observations for discussion with me in supervision.

There are several old patients seated around the walls of the day room. Apart from the observer no staff are present. One woman says, 'Someone has stolen my tin of biscuits, and we all know who it is!' She stares at one of the other women, who remains silent and seems unresponsive. One of the men, Mr H, is wearing a suit and tie. A carer comes in and says, 'Take your coat off Bill, it's too warm in here'. The carer leaves. Mr H then looks at a book of crossword puzzles. His wife, who is visiting and sitting alongside him, says crossly to him: 'Where is the pen? I'm not going to give you another pen if you're going to lose them!' Another woman, Mrs R, who appeared to be sleeping, opens her eyes and smiles at the observer saying, 'No more pens'. A different carer comes in and gives Mrs R a cup of tea, telling her not to spill it. Mrs R tries to put the cup and saucer on the floor. The carer tells her where to put it. The carer leaves. Mr H's wife tells him to drink his tea.

In this observation the general absence of the care staff was typical. Of course there are always practicalities to which staff need to attend and often minimal staffing, but I think a significant aspect that deters staff spending more time with their patients is the difficulty of feelings stirred from contact with patients suffering from dementia. The staff made occasional, brief appearances when their interventions were almost exclusively infantilising, often giving instructions as though to children. The infantilisation projectively evokes dependency in the patients who were treated as if they had almost no capacities. The patients' talk about theft is not uncommon, and suggests the dementia sufferers were unconsciously commenting on what they felt was lost through the incapacitating effects of their dementia, and stolen because of the way their carers treated them as though only the staff had capacities. The staff, faced with alarming reminders of their own possible futures and with little or no support, were vulnerable to projectively evoking feared helplessness and dependency in their patients, and thereby exacerbating the patients' incapacities.

In the next part of the observation Mrs R tries to get up out of her chair. The observer feels frightened Mrs R will fall. Mrs R flops back into her chair. Later she tries to get up again. She manages to stand up just as a carer comes in and says to her 'Sit down; you'll break your back!' Mrs R sits immediately. The observer is shocked. The carer leaves. Mrs R tries again. This time the observer feels like urging her on and wants to say, 'Come on, you can do it'. Another carer comes in and says to Mrs R 'Sit down or you'll fall!' Mrs R continues to try to stand up. The carer says impatiently 'Sit down! What's the matter with you!' Looking more closely, as though talking to a naughty child she says 'Oh you've gotten yourself wet'. The carer brings a wheelchair and takes Mrs R away (Terry, 2008).

Mrs R may have needed her carers to know her fears about a mind that was breaking apart. These fears were perhaps conveyed in the observer's and carer's counter-transference alarm Mrs R might fall and break her back. When the carer chastised Mrs R, the carer's projection of an infantile dependency protected her from the pain of identifying and suffering with a woman struggling to maintain some adult functioning.

Elliott Jaques (1965), in a seminal paper about fears of death which arise in mid-life, described what he found to be typical of the unconscious fear and experience of death which was depicted in a dream from one of his analytic patients. In the dream the patient was lying dead in a coffin, sliced up though connected with a thread of nerve to her brain. She was able to experience everything, knew she was dead but was unable to speak or move. This unconscious depiction of death is experienced in reality by people suffering from dementia, who are able to experience pain and distress, increasingly unable to communicate, reduced to appalling states of helplessness, and dependent on others for their every need. Jaques' formulations thus provide insight into how the development of increasing dependency, seen in its extreme in dementia, is particularly traumatic both for those suffering from dementia and their carers. The dementia comes to encapsulate an unconscious experience of death. Not surprisingly are people suffering from dementia sometimes referred to as the living dead.

Carers of people suffering from dementia can be recipients of powerful projections of unbearable feelings from their patients. Carers may therefore need to be able to bear not only their own fears of dependency and death, but also those same fears in their patients. This is a tall order, especially when carers are usually unsupported, and without help to appreciate that their feelings may bring some understanding about their patients' feelings.

An appreciation of the communicative aspects of projective identification contributes to various psychoanalytically informed non-verbal therapies which have been successfully developed for patients with dementia, including art, music, drama and dance therapy, and which are particularly helpful in the intermediate stage of dementia (Evans et al., 2004, 2020). Monitoring the counter-transference can guide therapists' understanding how patients are using these different non-verbal ways to communicate. Andrew Balfour has written about an experience of being in a group with patients suffering from dementia, when he found himself becoming more and more irritated with a woman who kept screaming incomprehensibly at the top of her voice. He said to her he felt she was very angry. For a few moments she became lucid and spoke movingly of her frustration (Balfour, 2007). Understanding may not be able to change disturbing behaviour, Balfour noted the woman was soon screaming again. However, having some understanding can make such behaviour more bearable for carers who may be exposed to it for many hours each day.

Balfour (2014) has written about developing therapeutic work with couples when one member of the couple is suffering from dementia. This work uses video recordings of couples in their homes to assist them to achieve better emotional contact, communication and understanding. I was fortunate to hear Balfour talk about this work with a couple he included in his article. The couple were videoed clearing out their fridge. The wife tended to stand aside waiting while her husband tried to do some of the clearing out. She became frustrated and angry about his failed attempts. Watching and then discussing the video recording with the therapist brought positive developments in the couple's relationship. Seeing the video may have helped the wife appreciate how standing aside watching her husband made it worse for him. Whether consciously or unconsciously, she would see how she was increasing her husband's helplessness. In other words she was projectively evoking her feared helplessness and dependency which worsened his helplessness. Her own rage and frustration perhaps gave some indication of her husband's unspoken feelings.

Helping carers become aware of the value of recognising their feelings as a source of understanding and communication with patients suffering from dementia is crucial. Essentially, this means reminding carers of the sensitivity and receptiveness that a mother or primary carer brings to caring for a baby who has no words. This is not to reduce patients suffering from dementia to infants, but to recognise that skills and sensitivities brought to parenting can be usefully drawn upon. These intuitive capacities can help carers find meaning in behaviour which otherwise might be dismissed as random or attention seeking. Especially in the presence of advanced dementia, if carers' fears are not recognised and supported, the fears can petrify these intuitive capacities. Such capacities contribute to being able to respond creatively and playfully to the wordless states of infants, and share enjoyment in pleasurable contact. These same capacities appear to petrify when in contact with those who portray our worst fears of dependency and death. Maggie Ellis and Arlene Astell (2010), have contributed to this field in developing an interactive technique that provides a means of helping carers to engage with patients suffering in advanced stages of dementia. These patients are often in prolonged states of dreadful inertia. The carer is encouraged to sit with a patient and wait for some bodily movement or reaction, and then simply to copy it each time it occurs. Ellis' and Astell's research shows their technique can restore a liveliness to those who seemed lost forever in withdrawn, inert states. The technique releases and supports carers' sensitivities and skills in order to help them re-establish contact, fun and hope with those who are severely incapacitated by dementia. The technique is reminiscent of Winnicott's (1971) insight about how the mother's capacity for mirroring promotes the infant's development.

Unlike infants, people suffering from dementia have long histories. Although dementia erodes and eventually erases the memories of those histories, carers can be important repositories for life stories and individual identities. It is therefore important that carers are encouraged to know the histories of their patients. Such knowledge can enhance their sensitivity when patients can no longer explain their feelings and behaviour. Margot Waddell (2000) writes about a woman suffering from dementia with little capacity left for verbal communication, who became distressed at the sudden noise of an approaching storm. Her daughter, because of knowledge of her mother's history, was able to offer much more than the reassurance that it was only a storm. She talked to her mother about how the noise was very likely a reminder of frightening aspects of her experiences in the Second World War. Her mother was much comforted by the daughter's words. Carers need support to know their patients because closeness to them can bring much anguish as the carers witness their patients' disintegration, and also need support to bear their patients' feelings about no longer knowing (Ramsay-Jones, 2019). Without adequate support, carers may try to protect themselves by remaining detached and ignorant of their patients' former lives.

Concluding Reflections

Reflecting on unconscious as well as conscious aspects of dementia reveals the depth of trauma suffered in the anticipation and later experience of extreme dependency in dementia. Carers are also exposed to a secondary or vicarious trauma, especially because of the resonance of extreme dependency with the unconscious experience of death. Mourning is central, mourning the losses that accompany ageing and incapacity, and ultimately the end of one's own life. People in the early stages of dementia may benefit from being helped to begin anticipatory mourning for the losses ahead. Family and friends may also need to be helped to mourn the experiences of increasing losses in loved ones who are suffering from dementia. These experiences of loss can be agonising when it means acknowledging losses that are irreversible. It is not uncommon for family members sometimes to become frustrated and angry about the dementia sufferer's memory lapses and constant repetitions, as though the lapses were deliberate or could be overcome. Whilst frustration is understandable, anger can be a protection against the painful knowledge that the loved one's forgetting is not by choice, but a symptom which will only worsen and eventually everything and everyone will be forgotten. I saw an elderly woman who became intensely irritable with her husband who was developing dementia. She wanted to leave him. She kept insisting she was fed up with her much older husband. In fact he was only a few years her senior but had become a frightening reminder of the vulnerabilities of being old. This woman became suicidally depressed. Her suicidal state projectively evoked fears of her own death in her carers, who were worried she would kill herself. Her fears of death were doubtless stirred by her husband's worsening dementia, and contributed to her discomfort of being with him.

For those of us who are approaching, or in old age, whatever our physical or mental capacities, death is inevitably on our agenda. Yet, in my experience, death was seldom present in the conscious agendas old people brought to therapy. More often, as will be explored in the next chapter in relation to the terminally ill, fears of death were denied. Denial of death obstructs mourning. Sinason's therapy with a patient suffering from dementia, shows how a therapist's capacity to give words for a patient's fears of death can bring relief and may enable mourning.

References

Balfour, A. (2007). Facts, phenomenology and psychoanalytic contributions to dementia care. In R. Davenhill (Ed.) *Looking into Later Life*. London: Karnac.

Balfour, A. (2014). Developing therapeutic couple work in dementia care – the living together with dementia project. *Psychoanalytic Psychotherapy*, 28 (3), 304–20.

Bick, E. (1968). The experience of skin in early object relations In E. Bott Spillius E. (ed.). *Melanie Klein To-day, Volume 1*. London: Routledge.

Ellis, M. & Astell, A. (2010). Communication and personhood in advanced dementia. *Healthcare Counselling and Psychotherapy Journal, 10* (3), 32–5.

Evans S. & Garner J. (Eds) (2004). *Talking Over the Years*. London: Brunner Routledge.

Evans, S., Garner, J. & Darnley-Smith, R. (Eds) (2020). *Psychodynamic Approaches to the Experience of Dementia*. London: Routledge.

Hess, N. (1987). King Lear and some anxieties of old age. *British Journal of Medical Psychology, 60*, 209–15.

Hess, N. (2004). Loneliness in old age: Klein and others. In S. Evans & J. Garner (Eds) (2004) *Talking Over the Years*. London: Brunner Routledge.

Hildebrand, P. (1995). *Beyond Mid-life Crisis: A Psychodynamic Approach to Ageing*. London: Sheldon Press.

Jaques, E. (1965). Death and the mid-life crisis. *International Journal of Psychoanalysis*, 46, 502–14.

Ramsay-Jones, E. (2019). *Holding Time: Human Need and Relationships in Dementia Care*. London: Free Association.

Sinason, V. (1992). *Mental Handicap and The Human Condition*. London: Free Association.

Symington, J. (1985). The survival function of primitive omnipotence. *International Journal of Psychoanalysis 66*, 481–7.

Terry, P (2008). *Counselling and Psychotherapy with Older People: A Psychodynamic Approach*. London: Palgrave Macmillan.

Waddell, M. (2000). Only connect: Development issues from early to later life. *Psychoanalytic Psychotherapy, 14*, 239–52.

Winnicott, D.W. (1971). *Playing and Reality* (London: Tavistock).

Chapter 3

Fears of Death and Fears of Dying

Introduction

It is commonplace for people to say they are not afraid of death but are afraid
of dying. My supervision of therapists working in a hospice with patients who
are terminally ill, developed my understanding of unconscious fears of death,
and enabled me to distinguish between unconscious fears of death and fears
of dying. I understood these fears in the counter-transferences of therapists
who were recipients of projective identifications about the fears. Although
I have already discussed counter-transference in the Introduction, there are
aspects of counter-transference to which Racker (2007) has drawn attention,
which I think helpful in thinking about the counter-transferences in this
chapter. Racker's formulations are that in the counter-transference the therapist may experience feelings similar to those which the patient believed were
the feelings of someone else, for example someone who may have abused the
patient. Racker describes this as a traditional view of counter-transference,
and calls it 'complementary' counter-transference. Or the therapist may
experience feelings similar to those which the patient experienced, such as in
being abused. Racker describes this as a more recent, wider view of counter-
transference, and calls it 'concordant' counter-transference. Racker thus clari-
fies how in the counter-transference we may identify with different aspects of
the patient's own feelings, or aspects of the feelings of significant others who
have become internal objects.

Fears of Dying

A therapist brought to supervision her therapy with a woman who was dying
in her early fifties. She was on an in-patient ward. The patient had a long history of physical illness. A few years previously there was a breakthrough in her
treatment when she began to experience better health. A short time later she
was discovered to have a terminal condition with little time left to live. The
patient was very frightened. Each time the therapist saw her patient she herself felt a 'heart racing sense of panic'. She felt desperate to relieve the patient's

DOI: 10.4324/9781003319719-6

fear. She decided to use techniques such as mindfulness to try to help the patient manage her fear. The medical staff were impatient with her patient. The patient had been on the ward a bit longer than usual, and they thought she was well enough to be treated from home. In a ward round the consultant said that 'of course they could not put themselves in her shoes but…'. The patient's husband had said to her that at least she knew when she was likely to die. She described a 'tough love' mother.

This snapshot of the patient's mother suggests she offered poor containment for her daughter's vulnerable feelings. She was probably not a mother on whom this woman could depend, but became an internal object who insisted on toughness and condemned helplessness. I suspect this internal tough mother had not much time for her daughter's fears; nor it seems did her husband or the medical staff. The impatience of the medical staff suggests they indeed had some inkling of being in her shoes but couldn't bear it. Her therapist's heart racing panic gives some indication of how unbearable her patient's fears felt in the therapist's identification with the patient in the counter-transference. Martindale (2007) understands fears of dying 'reawaken' fears of dependency from early failures in the dependency relationship. For this patient fears of dependency seem linked to a fear that no-one would want to care for her in her dying state. These fears were made real by projective identification and can be seen in the medical staff's somewhat atypical impatience to discharge her. The husband seemed to be similarly impatient with her. The staff and husband seemed identified with a counter-transference which brought about enactments of likely early failures in the patient's dependency relationship. When her therapist reached for behavioural techniques to alleviate the patient's panic, the therapist's departure from her usual psychodynamic approach suggests a counter-transference enactment, in which by abandoning her usual containment it was as though she could no longer bear the intensity of the patient's projections. Gavin Ivey (2015) describes how a dynamic therapist is vulnerable to such enactments when in the counter-transference there is a pressure to introduce active interventions. He discusses how psychoanalytic or psychodynamic containment already encompasses important elements of mindfulness techniques. He illustrates how, during a dynamic therapy, the introduction of mindfulness techniques may involve an enactment. He stresses the importance of therapists reflecting upon the counter-transference before making such alterations in their approach.

As I have indicated, it is important also to consider projections from a punitive superego. Such superego admonitions are implicit in the glimpses of this patient's past and present life, for example in the tough mother, harsh sounding husband, and impatient medical staff. The therapist's superego, evoked in her counter-transference, may have influenced abandoning her psychodynamic approach. This kind of superego may have contributed to the patient's distress by making her feel guilty about feeling fearful and helpless, and may have been projectively evoked in others. As discussed in the previous chapter, fears of dependency may likely lead to seeking refuge in a strong, ruthless superego to hold the self together.

A therapist was seeing a woman in her sixties whose somewhat older husband was a patient of the hospice. Her husband had become quarrelsome and verbally abusive. The patient told the therapist she planned to leave her husband, but could not do so when he was diagnosed with an incurable Motor Neurone Disease. He was no longer allowed to drive their car. She described driving him on a long car journey during which he continually shouted abuse at her. She stopped the car and burst into tears. She said she felt trapped because she was unable to leave him. Her therapist found herself hoping the patient would leave the husband. At a later session her patient reported the husband saying he thought the therapy was helping her, and he wondered if he should have therapy too. She then told the therapist her husband had been adopted at an early age. He was told repeatedly by his adoptive parents how special he was, because he was specially chosen by them. He was a perfectionist and had achieved a successful professional career.

Suffering from a Motor Neurone Disease, this man faced a long, lingering death. His intact mind would eventually be trapped in a body no longer able to function. He would become unable to speak, eat or eventually breathe. I suspect that signs of his degenerative condition already affected him before the formal diagnosis; and prompted unconscious fears of becoming dependent and being abandoned, which were revived from his infancy. In the account of his adoption, as so often happens, mourning was discouraged (Kirschner, 2007). Instead he was encouraged to feel specially chosen. I think it was again difficult for him to mourn his degenerative illness and death. In his abusive behaviour he projectively evoked feelings in his wife which brought about an enactment of the feared abandonment. The result was that she was on the brink of leaving him before his diagnosis was known. The therapist was inclined to identify with the wife's criticisms of the husband and the wish to abandon him. Importantly the therapist did not discharge her countertransference feelings into some kind of action, for example by advising her patient to leave her husband. Instead, her reflectiveness and containment enabled her patient to develop an understanding of her husband's fears, especially as they were probably revived from his early adoption. The husband's perfectionism and high achievement indicates a harsh superego with which he held himself together, and which probably exacerbated his distress about increasing debility.

The gradual decline in capacities in Multiple Sclerosis or Motor Neurone Disease is resonant with aspects of dementia, discussed in the previous chapter in relation to the unconscious experience and fear of death. The experience in the dream of Jaques' patient being able to experience pain and distress but unable to communicate, also becomes real for those who suffer incurable illnesses like Motor Neurone Disease or Multiple Sclerosis, and who are eventually unable to express their needs. Illnesses like these are often reduced to acronyms like MND or MS, which easily slip off the tongue in a way that can assist not thinking about the horrific experiences they inflict. Although Jaques links the dream image to the fear of death it is more evocative of a fear of dying because it captures the dread of a failed dependency.

A therapist presented a man of just 41 years who, as a result of Multiple Sclerosis, was confined to a wheelchair with just a few remaining capacities, which were diminishing almost daily. The therapist worried because she found herself feeling in agreement with her patient's expressed wish he would die to end his suffering. I was surprised at how little she knew about his life. She said she felt uncomfortable asking him any questions about his life. It seemed she and her patient could only think about his wish to end his life. When her patient later talked more about his life, he revealed poor relationships with both parents, which seemed related to his decision not to have children. He recalled long periods in his teens when his mother was absent because of illness. I thought this could indicate a screen memory (Freud, 1899) for earlier maternal absence. Freud thought certain memories were unconsciously a screen, some for earlier memories and some for later memories, which were unmanageable consciously and were repressed. Undoubtedly illnesses like Multiple Sclerosis are horribly difficult to bear but they are likely to be even more unbearable when needs have not been adequately met in the early dependency relationship, which leaves a dread of becoming dependent again. The therapist's identification with her patient's wish he would die, could lead to an enactment in the counter-transference of his experience about feeling no-one could bear his dependency needs.

In contrast to the previous patient who seemed only to want to think about his wish to die, this next vignette describes a patient who seemed preoccupied with the past. A woman in her mid-fifties, who was under the care of a hospice, was referred for therapy. She was at the time still managing to live on her own. Her therapist mentioned, almost in passing, that she had 'MS', and went on to talk enthusiastically about the patient's keen interest in exploring aspects of her early life. I reminded him about her Multiple Sclerosis. I suggested perhaps the preoccupation with looking backwards in time might be taking them both away from a difficult present. When the therapist again discussed the patient he told me he asked her more about her illness. He discovered she had a rare form of Multiple Sclerosis which meant she could die at any time. She started talking about how hard it was being alone. She blamed herself for causing her illness, believing it was the result of her anger with her partner after they separated. She described a harrowing relationship with her sister who was often cruel to her. I thought what was revealed was a cruel superego blaming her for her loneliness and having Multiple Sclerosis.

When the nature of this patient's Multiple Sclerosis and the possible imminence of death came to light, the patient admitted she thought about dying every day. This meant the matter of how long she might live and her priorities in the remaining time, could then be addressed. Whilst supervising therapy with those who are terminally ill, I have found that the patient's prognosis and how long the patient expects to live, are sometimes unknown, not explored or discussed. Undoubtedly these are difficult questions but, as Dr Atul Gawande (2014) has confirmed, these questions are infrequently addressed with those who are terminally ill. Gawande discusses how hard it is for doctors to acknowledge the limits of the relentless treatments they feel obliged to offer terminally ill patients. He found there is often a great deal of relief when patients are asked how much time they think they have left, and when they are prompted to think about their priorities in the time remaining. He also observed some patients were not able to talk about these issues, but might benefit from psychotherapeutic help in order to do so.

Fears of Death

Fears of death are much more difficult to detect, as indicated, such fears are often consciously denied and as the following vignettes illustrate unconscious fears of death are manifest in elusive disguises in the conscious material and in the counter-transference.

I was asked to see a man in his early seventies, who was a patient in a specialist mental health service for older people. He was discharged to the day hospital from an in-patient ward where he had been admitted because of a suicide attempt. I was told he still had occasional thoughts of suicide, but was no longer regarded as an active suicide risk. The staff in the day hospital had reached an impasse with him. He was physically well, had retired on a substantial pension, and lived with his wife in a fine house. He had been keenly involved in the care of the garden. He had been a regular golfer at the local club, where he had friends with whom he socialised. But no longer. His previously active life had come to a standstill. He sat in an armchair at home or the day hospital, unwilling to do anything. He agreed to see me, though he soon made it clear he felt no need of my help. He offered little and gave cryptic answers to questions about his life. I quickly came to appreciate the day hospital staff's frustration.

He attended a second appointment and, on further questioning, spoke a bit about his golfing. The last time he played golf one of his friends had a heart attack on the putting green, and died in front of him. He never returned to the golf course. Probably somewhat precipitately and reflecting my irritation with him, I interpreted that I thought he was afraid of having a stroke like his friend, and was fearful any exertion might kill him, so he resolved to do nothing. He dismissed such fears with much contempt. Towards the end of this meeting he talked in a way which implied he might try to kill himself at a nearby level rail crossing, without admitting that was his intention. I was left worried it was just what he would do, and alerted the day hospital staff. When they later did a risk assessment at his home, he denied all such thoughts. He refused to see me again.

In my interpretation about his fears of death I failed to address, but instead enacted, a harsh superego projectively evoked in the counter-transference. This suggests a sadistic superego doubtless linked with this patient's depression, and unwillingness to acknowledge his fears. I felt a persecuting guilt about not stopping him from leaving the unit when I felt he was at risk of killing himself. Later, I realised I had not appreciated the patient's unconscious communication of his persecuting guilt about his helplessness to stop his friend dying. When I worried he would kill himself, he was also probably evoking his unconscious fears of death, but on reflection what seemed paramount was a persecuting guilt about not saving his friend's life, and that guilt probably contributed to his suicidal feelings.

A therapist brought concerns to supervision about her patient who was terminally ill. The patient suffered a great deal from a deteriorating physical state and was an in-patient. For some time she kept expressing a wish to die. The therapist told me she was worried about safeguarding issues in relation to this woman's husband, who was her sole carer. She said some of the nurses on the ward also voiced concerns about the woman's husband. When I explored the nature of the worries, the therapist was hard pressed to describe what it was that worried her and the nurses. Although there had been recent arguments between the couple, there was no evidence of physical abuse. Her patient spoke of how well her husband cared for her, and how they enjoyed watching television together. The patient died a little time later. The therapist was extremely upset, and puzzled about how much more affected she had been by the death of this patient, in contrast to deaths of other patients with whom she'd worked.

To the therapist and nurses there seemed a threat of injury or death of the patient from her husband. There was no substantial evidence for this threat, but this woman would soon die from a terminal illness. In contrast to this patient's understandable longing to die to end her suffering, the safeguarding concerns evoked in the therapist's and nurses' counter-transference, indicate the patient's unconscious fears of death. A further aspect of this projective process was later apparent in the extreme grief the therapist felt about her patient's death. The patient's wish to live was split off and projectively evoked in the therapist. In her anguished dying, the patient could not manage a more ambivalent position of wanting to die and wanting to live.

A therapist brought an old male patient who was dying from two different forms of cancer. He complained of feeling claustrophobic in the counselling room, and said 'there was no way out' of the hospice. He recalled an experience when he was just a boy playing a game with an older sibling. In the game he was nearly suffocated by having a pillow held over his face for too long. The therapist felt shocked and frightened by the story. The patient's fears of death were near to consciousness, but it was located at a much earlier time in his life when he was a boy, and nearly suffocated. In the therapist's counter-transference, she was given a glimpse of how frightened her patient felt in the present about his impending death, which was his only way out of the hospice.

Another therapist was asked to see a terminally ill patient for an assessment for therapy in the patient's home because, though the patient requested therapy, he refused to go to the hospice. When the therapist met the man he felt alarmed that he would be assaulted, not so much from what the man said, but more in response to being with him. The therapist was shaken by the experience, and troubled about why he had become fearful for his own survival. The therapist's own fears of death were evoked in the counter-transference, which reveal his patient's unconscious fears. Those fears doubtless contributed to the patient's reluctance to go to the hospice, which would have meant acknowledging his dying condition.

Ending Therapy

Drawing therapy to a close is often difficult especially because those who seek therapy so frequently bring painful experiences of loss. Ending with those who are dying can be very hard as the following vignette illustrates.

A therapist brings to supervision a young woman in her thirties suffering from a terminal illness, and currently being treated with a gruelling chemotherapy programme. The therapist wonders how long she should see her patient for. I wonder how long her patient expects to live. A few months later, the therapist tells me her patient, who has been longing for the end of the chemotherapy, has now been told she will have to remain on chemotherapy until she dies. The chemotherapy will not cure her illness, but might extend her life. She finds the side effects dreadful to bear. I wonder why she puts up with it. Could it not be preferable to put a stop to this treatment which she finds so distressing? The therapist says those thoughts also passed through her mind. I say it could be helpful to put such thoughts into words. A few weeks later, I hear about a session in which the therapist and her patient seem nearer to talking about the reality of the patient's death. Again I raise the question of setting an ending date saying, as I usually do, that it doesn't matter quite what date is agreed but it seems to me important it is addressed.

Several weeks later the therapist admits she is struggling to raise ending of the therapy, particularly because the patient feels so unsupported by her family. The contact the therapist had with her patient's parents indicated they could not manage their daughter's dying. I remind the therapist it is the discussion about ending which is important, the acknowledgment that time and life are finite.

The next month I hear the patient has been given a deadline she was told she has no more than a year to live. She talks of how she has to keep things light and humorous for her friends, whom she describes as heartless. I was reminded of accounts of her parents' insensitivity to her distress, which confirm her fear no-one, including her therapist, can bear to know about her feelings.

She jokes with her therapist that at least death will mean she no longer has to struggle to find a partner and happiness. She talks more about a psychiatric history which suggests she has suffered a considerable time with depression, which she has tried to self medicate in different ways. I notice in the accounts of the sessions, it is as though the patient has plenty of time in the way she talks of projects she is trying to pursue. She is in a debilitated state, and her efforts to pursue these projects seem tormenting.

Six months after I first raised the question of an ending, the therapist discusses it with her patient. In response the patient says she would like to continue until she dies, but she can appreciate there must be questions of resources for therapy, and it may not be possible. The therapist assures her it is not a question of resources, but it is important for them to think about ending. A few weeks later the therapist comes saying how guilty she feels because she and her patient have still not agreed an ending date. She describes a recent session in which her patient is painfully reflecting on what she has missed out on in her life, and which will now be impossible. Despite these regrets, she is able to acknowledge some of her considerable achievements. There is a poignant sadness. The patient and therapist are engaged in the crucial work of mourning the end of her life.

I believe this movement into mourning was enabled by confronting the end of the therapeutic relationship. Setting an ending date is an issue which comes up particularly in therapy with those who are suffering in old age and, or terminally ill. I have argued elsewhere (Terry, 2008) that difficulties experienced by therapists in ending with old patients, can reflect how the therapists' own fears of death are projectively evoked by their elderly patients. To raise the ending of therapy with someone who is dying is undoubtedly difficult, but doing so can bring an opportunity in the here-and-now of the therapeutic relationship, for the finiteness of life and time to be mourned with other losses including the ending of one's own life. If an ending to the therapy is not addressed, it can confirm an apprehension that the emotional experience of such losses cannot be borne by the patient or the therapist. Therapist and patient together facing the ending of their relationship, may bring some hope that what may seem unthinkable about death can be faced. I believe it is important to reflect on the counter-transference involved in a reluctance to address an ending to the therapy. There are no hard and fast strictures about what to decide in these distressing end of life tragedies. Alongside reflection on the counter-transference, considerations of the dying person's particular life experiences, emotional resources and support need to guide the therapist.

Concluding Reflections on Death and Dying

Freud wrote about our attitude towards death in 'Thoughts for the Times on War and Death' in 1915, six months after the outbreak of the First World War. He had two sons fighting in the war. At this time he was also drafting his paper about mourning and melancholia, ideas for which had first been sketched a year after his father's death, nineteen years earlier. In his thoughts about war and death, Freud described a ubiquitous denial of death, which was challenged at times of war because there were so many deaths. He wrote it is 'impossible to imagine our own death; and whenever we attempt to do so we can perceive that we are in fact still present as spectators ... at bottom no-one believes in his own death ... in the unconscious everyone of us is convinced of his own immortality' (Freud, 1915, p. 289).

Freud left us with a conundrum of the unthinkableness of death and the diminishing of our lives by denial of death.

In Klein's paper 'On the Sense of Loneliness' (1963), drafted only a few months before she died, her editors comment she seems to have a premonition of her death. She wrote about fears of death which 'play a part in loneliness' and how earliest fears about one's death arise in infancy during the mother's absences, when the 'feeling that she is lost is equivalent to the fear of her death'. As a result of introjection, 'the death of the external mother means the loss of the internal good object as well, and this reinforces the infant's fear of his own death' (p. 304). In Klein's formulation the self is still present. Similarly, in the image which Jaques describes as the unconscious experience of death in the patient's dream, the self is still present. There have been relatively few references to unconscious fears of death in psychoanalytic writings. It seems Freud's 1915 insight about the denial of death was not pursued until 2004 by Franco De Masi in his book *Making Death Thinkable*. De Masi describes the anticipation of death as a trauma to the mind like no other trauma, because it represents nothingness, the loss of self. Perhaps the unthinkableness of death accounts for the reluctance of Freud's followers to pursue his insight; and may also explain why detection of fears of death in the counter-transference can be difficult, and why it can sometimes be hard to set an ending date for those who are old or terminally ill. By contrast fears of dying are more accessible, because in fears of dying the self still exists though with fears of being let down and abandoned when dependent and in need.

Fears of death were powerfully conveyed to me on an occasion after supervising at the hospice. During the day I had been troubled by some pain in my chest which I thought due to indigestion. On my journey home the pain persisted. I became alarmed I might be having a heart attack, and went to an Accident and Emergency department. Following an investigation I was given the all clear and discharged, and the pain disappeared. I recalled a supervision meeting during the day with a therapist, who had only recently begun working in the hospice. The therapist was troubled by an incident on the in-patient ward. She had started 'popping in' on patients to chat to them, without the patients having been referred to the counselling service. She thought this could be a way of making herself known on the ward. She brought a recent incident when she popped in to see a patient. The patient was with some members of his family. While she was there the patient suddenly burst into tears saying how frightened he was about dying. The therapist felt shocked and couldn't think of anything to say. She was deeply upset about being struck dumb. We discussed how in these circumstances she was neither a friend, family member nor the patient's therapist, and how important it was to have a professional role to help contain and manage the patient's, and our own, feelings. It is not uncommon, if a friend or family witnesses the death of a loved one, for that person to become afraid of dying. In retrospect, my impression was that without some protection of professional boundaries, the therapist was unable to keep some balance between being open to the patient's projections, at the same as being able to step back to think about the patient's fear of death. Instead the therapist became petrified with fear herself. After this supervision session in a 'parallel process' (Mattison, 1975) I became identified with my supervisee's palpable and uncontained fear of death.

References

De Masi, F. (2004). *Making Death Thinkable.* London: Free Association.

Freud, S. (1899). Screen memories. *The Standard Edition of the Complete Psychological Works of Sigmund Freud*, III, 299–322.

Freud, S. (1915). Thoughts for the times on war and death. *The Standard Edition of the Complete Psychological Works of Sigmund Freud, XIV*, 273–300.

Gawande, A. (2014). *Being Mortal.* London: Profile Books.

Ivey, G. (2011). Bion's therapeutic applications. *Psychoanalytic Psychotherapy, 25*, 92–104.

Ivey, G. (2015). The mindfulness status of psychoanalytic psychotherapy. *Psychoanalytic Psychotherapy, 29* (4), 382–98.

Jaques, E. (1965). Death and the mid-life crisis. *The International Journal of Psychoanalysis, 46*, 502–14.

Kirschner, D. (2007). Sometimes a fatal quest: Losses in adoption. In B. Willock, L. Bohm & R. Curtis (Eds) *On Deaths and Endings* (pp. 161–8). London: Routledge.

Klein, M. (1963/1975). On the sense of loneliness. In R. Money-Kirle, B. Joseph, E. O'Shaughnessy & H. Segal (Eds) *Envy and Gratitude and Other Works* (pp. 300–13). London: Hogarth Press.

Martindale, B. (2007). Resilience and vulnerability in later life. *British Journal of Psychotherapy, 23* (2), 205–16.

Mattinson, J. (1975). *The Reflection Process in Casework Supervision.* London: Institute of Martial Studies, The Tavistock Institute of Human Relations.

Racker, H. (2007). The meanings and uses of countertransference. *The Psychoanalytic Quarterly, 76* (3), 725–77.

Terry, P. (2008). *Counselling and Psychotherapy with Older People: A Psychodynamic Approach.* London: Palgrave Macmillan.

Part III

Psychosis

Chapter 4

Violence and Psychosis

Introduction

My experience of working in a Psychiatric Intensive Care Unit revealed to me how someone suffering from psychosis and vulnerable to being violent may use projective identification to convey profound fears in physical violence. The Unit comprised two secure wards, one acute and one rehabilitation ward. There were seven patients on each ward. The patients were male, suffering from paranoid schizophrenia and had committed, or were regarded as at risk of committing, acts of violence. Soon after my appointment I was asked to conduct an assessment with R, a white man who was in his thirties. He had a long psychiatric history. He was admitted to the ward because he grievously assaulted another man, who was a passer-by and a stranger to him. At the time it seemed R believed the man was part of a conspiracy against him. He had been on the ward for some months while he awaited the outcome of court deliberations about his future. He was no longer explicitly delusional. At ward rounds I had observed that R presented himself with an attitude of butter-wouldn't-melt-in-his-mouth innocence. He spoke of some remorse about what he had done, but more as though he thought this was what was expected of him rather than what he felt. He seemed devoid of any feelings for his victim, uncomprehending about the gravity of his crime, and bewildered that he might be sentenced to spend a long time in high security accommodation. He said he was writing about his life, and offered to show his story to the consultant psychiatrist, somewhat coyly almost as though she was a prospective publisher. Apparently he had only written about his life up to the time of the assault, which was not mentioned.

In the assessment interview R made it clear he believed he didn't need any psychological help, and he kept the meeting brief. In a hasty sketch of his life he said his childhood had been idyllic, and added as an afterthought that his mother liked her sherry. He said his mother had died two years previously. Her death had 'hit him like a ton of bricks'. A thick set fellow, I felt R was like a menacing bouncer. I was relieved when he cut the interview short. Later, I reflected on how in his assault on the stranger R had passed on his

DOI: 10.4324/9781003319719-8

experience of being hit like a ton of bricks. The incident illustrated the use of projective identification in a violent enactment. R made the stranger feel how he himself felt but discharged the feelings in a physical assault.

Violence and Projective Identification

In a chapter titled 'The use of the body' from the book *Psychoanalytic Understanding of Violence and Suicide*, Peter Fonagy and Mary Target link violence with early problems in containment. They describe containment as the capacity of the mother or primary caregiver 'to demonstrate to the child that she thinks of him or her as an intentional being whose behaviour is driven by thoughts, feelings, beliefs and desires' (Fonagy & Target 1999, p.54); and they argue that failures in this maternal capacity lead to a fragile sense of self which violent behaviour is aimed at protecting. They write 'Where a patient cannot easily conceive of an object at a psychological level, he may seek identifications or create representations of mental states via the body, and this can predispose to acts of physical violence directed at himself or others' (1999, p.63).

I came to see that as a result of early problems in containment there may not develop an internal capacity for processing painful emotional experience. Consequently, violence may reflect the use of projective identification to evacuate unbearable emotional pain. It is as though a sense of containment can only be experienced by seeing physical evidence of the pain in the other person's body. R experienced the shock and grief about his mother's death like an assault on his body and forced that experience into a stranger. This can also be understood as a symbolic-concrete retaliation against his mother whom he may have experienced as a stranger when she became drunk with her sherry (William Halton, personal communication).

Fear of Separateness and Fear of Closeness

Mary Brownescombe Heller (2003) has written about issues of containment with a violent borderline female patient. She describes a session with her patient in which there was a rare moment of emotional contact between them. At the end of the session just as the patient was about to leave the consulting room she suddenly, with considerable force, slapped the therapist across the face. Following some real emotional connection in the session, the pain of leaving the therapist was too hard to bear. The patient needed the therapist to feel her shock and pain at separation in a physical way. The projective process not only evacuated and communicated the patient's emotional state, it also attempted to overcome the pain of separateness. The phantasy of forcing her shocked and hurt self into the therapist merged the patient with her therapist.

Fonagy & Target (1999) link difficulties in achieving a separate autonomous identity also with early problems in containment between mother and infant. As discussed in Chapter 2, Bick (1968) drew attention to how early problems in containment can lead to premature ways of trying to hold the self together, but leave a dread of unintegration, of falling to pieces. The dread of unintegration for example can lead to relying on physical musculature to try to steel oneself against this dread, or to creating omnipotent structures in the mind. Studies of pathological and psychotic organizations in the mind, particularly by John Steiner (1993), reveal underlying and complex webs of projective identification that bind a fragile self together. External figures, who in phantasy are recipients of projected parts of the self, are internalised often as cohesive, tight knit gangs. Steiner describes how the mind can be dominated by psychotic and pathological organisations. He sees the organisations as a 'psychic retreat' from a dread of paranoid schizoid fragmentation or depressive pain. A talion reaction to this omnipotent use of projective identification, which includes the phantasy of being able to take over someone else's mind, can lead to a belief of being taken over by external voices or figures who are felt to be controlling one's thoughts and actions. It seems that both the slap of Brownescombe Heller's patient and R's 'ton of bricks' attack may reflect a use of projective identification in a violent enactment because of overwhelming anxieties that were stirred by separation.

Fear of closeness is the other side of a conflict which may oscillate with fear of separateness. Mervin Glasser who worked with violent patients, developed the concept of a 'core complex' that describes 'an intense longing for indissoluble union with the object, typically the mother, which leaves the individual at the same time, with a fear of being merged and annihilated'(Perelberg 1999, p.3). Although closeness may be wanted to overcome fears of abandonment and separateness, it can bring fears of merger and death. Fear of merger may indicate the projection of a need to hold onto and control someone. Such a need to control the other will be all the more intense when there is a dread of fragmentation or unintegration, and give the need to control a life and death kind of tenacity. This intense need to control in its projected form may then be experienced as a deadly threat. The fear of merger may result from problems in early childhood when the infant received massive projections from a mother, who herself probably lacked containment. Psychoanalytic studies of suicide reveal an unconscious phantasy in which killing oneself is seen as an attempt to free the self from being merged with a persecutory, engulfing or abandoning maternal figure. The maternal figure is concretely identified with the pain in the physical body. Killing the body is meant to free the self from this persecuting merger, in order for the self to merge with an idealized mother in a painless state of bliss (Campbell & Hale 1991, 2017).

S, a young white male in his early twenties, had a long history of admissions to the Psychiatric Unit. He was an only child, his father left him and his mother when S was still an infant. As an adult S tried but could not manage to live independently from his mother. An incident which terrified his mother occurred when S, deluded and aggressive, held her hostage and threatened to rape her. This brief and traumatic episode, in a bodily way captures the terror of engulfment which S forcibly expelled into his mother. S was guarded and suspicious on the acute ward. He was reluctant to divulge his thoughts and there was some worry that he might be experiencing command hallucinations. When I saw him for an assessment he was sullen and unwilling to speak. After a few minutes he asked to leave. I said if he changed his mind I would see him again. Some weeks later, it seemed that the medication had some effect, his guardedness and suspiciousness eased and he was transferred to the rehabilitation ward. I was told that he wanted to see me. I offered another appointment. Just before the appointment I saw S in the dayroom. I noticed, somewhat uncomfortably, he still looked rather menacing and suspicious. He came into the consulting room, closed the door and locked it from the inside. He declined to sit in a chair adjacent to me. Instead he chose the other chair which was immediately opposite to me. I felt frightened about the locked door, and nervous under S's piercing gaze. I was unsure what to do. I decided to wait. S's features gradually softened a little. He started speaking. He talked in a rambling, incoherent way. I felt confused, and for some time found it hard to think. Finally, I said that I thought that he felt in pieces, and was trying to hold himself together. This seemed to make some connection with him. He said he would like to see me again next week. I spent the intervening week worrying about what to do if he locked the door again, without reaching any conclusion. When S came to the next appointment he was visibly more relaxed, did not lock the door and sat in the chair adjacent to me. In retrospect, in relation to him locking the door I should have taken some precautions before the next meeting, instead of denying the risk of violence. I was identified with the institutional denial of violence which had kept the internal lock on the door.

I think an important aspect of S's locking me in the room with him, was to let me know something of his fear of being trapped inside someone else, probably his mother. During the interview I was also frightened and confused by his fragmented state of mind. When I could put some thoughts into words, he probably felt some relief that I could separate myself enough from him to begin to think about him. My counter-transference fears of being trapped or about a confusing, fragmented mind conveyed S's oscillation between the fears of closeness or separateness.

To summarise, fears of closeness and fears of separateness in these patients seem linked to an underlying dread of unintegration or fragmentation. These fears are essentially terrors of annihilation. Violence may attempt to resolve fears about separateness by merger, which may then stir fears of closeness; or violence may attempt to resolve fears of closeness by withdrawal, which may then stir fears of separateness. Hence for these patients there can be a dynamic oscillation between these fears, and a predilection to use violence as a means of evacuating the underlying dread of annihilation.

The Importance of Father or a Third Figure

P is an Afro Caribbean man who was in his late thirties when I saw him on the acute ward. He had his first breakdown when he was just 17 years of age and at college. In the following 13 years he had 19 admissions. His psychotic episodes, as for many of the patients in the unit, were exacerbated and perhaps precipitated by drug and alcohol abuse. At the first interview he was pleased to see me and talk about his life. He was fluent and articulate, but talked continuously and in a meandering way, moving from one fragmented thought to another without any apparent connection. I found him hard to follow. I couldn't make much sense of what he was telling me. After some time, I became aware of some oblique references to colour and race which were inserted in his obscure monologue. I interrupted him to acknowledge the colour and racial differences between us, and what I felt might be some of his worries about these differences. This interpretation had a dramatic effect. He looked me in the eye and spoke directly to me. For the remainder of the interview he talked in a way I could follow. Movingly, he told me his father could not find the time to spend with him, and couldn't understand him. He spoke about the importance of physical contact. He said when he arrived in the unit he was shattered, but one of the nurses touched him and it was a great help. I think when he arrived at his interview with me he felt in pieces. I quickly became a father who didn't understand him. I think he was letting me know that by my interpretation, and perhaps by taking the time to try to understand him, he felt touched by the contact with me, which helped him to gather himself together and feel more integrated.

My interpretation was helpful because it articulated in a quite physical way some of the differences between P and myself. At that moment I extricated myself from a powerful projection of an uncomprehending father transference, whereby I was projectively merged with P. Giving words to our separateness, embodied in our different racial identities, enabled a contact between us as two separate people. P's reference to his father's absence was significant, especially because it usually falls to father, or a third figure, to help mother and infant separate, and help mother disentangle herself from the infant's or child's projections.

The Portman Clinic in London offers specialist psychoanalytic therapy for people seeking help because of their violence. At the clinic's 70th Anniversary Conference titled 'Who's afraid of whom?', Don Campbell gave a paper in which he described 'now moments' between patient and therapist. As an illustration he recalled some of his early work with a man who had a history of violence. During a discussion with his colleagues at the Portman, Campbell realized that he had joined in with a 'delusion' in which he and his patient denied the patient's propensity for violence. This realization led Campbell to remove a heavy ashtray he'd left on the desk in his office, before his next session with the patient. As Campbell wryly pointed out the use of an ashtray shows how long ago it was. At the session, the patient said in a threatening and triumphant voice 'I notice you've removed the ashtray!' This was the 'now moment', a moment of an emotional frisson in the session. Such moments may also occur outside the session, for example when a therapist might unexpectedly encounter a patient in a supermarket or a cinema queue. Campbell said that for some time he felt more at risk and frightened as a result of stirring the patient's paranoid fantasies by the removal of the ashtray.

My understanding of this 'now moment' is that it occurred because of the intervention of a third party. Campbell's colleagues' discussion with him about the patient, helped Campbell disentangle himself from the delusions of the transference and counter-transference. In other words he was able to disentangle himself from projective processes, in which he was taken over and became identified with a psychotic part of the patient's mind, which denied the patient's violence. The intervention of the third party meant that at least for a while Campbell was freed from those projections; and so too perhaps the patient who, Campbell reported, spoke to him for the first time in a direct way. The language of the patient, that he 'had noticed' the therapist, suggests an observing, third position, much as Campbell's colleagues offered a third perspective. I see the 'now moment' as a moment of real contact between two separate individuals, who were not at that moment in a merged state, glued together by projective identification. When, in a now moment it is as though therapist and patient metaphorically or actually bump into one another, the frisson of the reality in the contact occurs because of the simultaneous, and often unwelcome realization, of the separateness of the other. Genuine intimacy can only occur from a recognition of separateness (Fisher & Ruszczynski, 1995), which for violent and psychotic patients may bring dreads that projective identification tries to escape.

Although Campbell felt more at risk with his patient, he wasn't attacked, and indeed in 70 years of the Portman Clinic's history, there were remarkably few instances of violence. What contributes to this containment of violence is evident in Campbell's illustration of the regular discussions with colleagues about each others' work. The colleagues function as third figures supporting the therapist and patient, and who are like a helpful father, or significant other supporting mother and infant against dangers of merger. At the same time this third figure enables therapist and patient to achieve a closeness which comes from recognising separateness. A recurring theme reported in work with violent patients is an absent or ineffective father. Rosine Jozef Pereleberg (1999), who has edited a book of work from a research project studying the analyses of violent patients, writes in her introduction about the recurring theme in these analyses of the importance of the role of the father:

> 'The role of the father in helping the child to develop a space in which he can see himself as separate from the mother is a theme that permeates this

book. The absence of the father or his violence makes things worse as he is not available to present the child with the experience of a positive relationship between the parental couple. As a result he does not facilitate the child's capacity to experience himself in relation to his objects nor does he offer an alternative to the phantasies of fusion with a mother'.

(Pereleberg 1999, pp. 7–8)

Pereleberg comments how the research group in the project was like a father supporting analysts and patients, particularly helping the patients to feel 'less isolated and threatened' when alone with the analyst in the consulting room. Pereleberg's words echo those of Caper (1999) who understands that the therapist manages to disentangle him or herself from the patient's projections because of a relationship in the mind to psychoanalysis, which functions like the relationship mother has with father or other third figure which helps her to disentangle herself from her infant's projections, a theme which is discussed further in Chapter 7.

Concluding Reflections

In accounts of therapy with people suffering from their violence, the need for mourning is a recurring theme. Arthur Hyatt Williams (1998), one of the first psychoanalysts to work in prisons, in a book about his life's work *Cruelty, Violence and Murder* stresses the need for violent offenders to mourn. He explains they need to mourn the violent fantasies, and much more difficult to mourn the consequences of actual violence and murder. Klein (1940) understood that experiences of mourning unconsciously resonate with early experiences of separation from the mother. If there were problems in containment, then the threat of the loss of the mother can feel catastrophic, because there is little inner sense of containment to manage fears of separateness. Mourning can thus be blocked because a capacity for separateness is a precondition for being able to mourn.

An illustration of how mourning can be associated with terrors of annihilation occurred with a patient L. I was asked to see L, an Afro Caribbean who was on the rehabilitation ward. He was then in his late thirties, with a long history of psychotic illness. He often suffered from bizarre delusions about his body, and would go to Accident and Emergency insisting on tests and scans. When I saw him, he had a friendly and cheerful demeanour, was willing to see me but said he didn't feel he needed my help. He told me about a life of hardship and disappointment, although as a young man he felt a lot of promise about his life ahead. He had good memories of school where he had done well and of being in the Boys Brigade. Later he said he fell into bad company, but did not elaborate. He said that he had had 23 different jobs. The third time I saw L he brought a dream. He said it was his first dream for a long time. In the dream he was on a railway station with lots of luggage. He looked around and suddenly all the luggage had disappeared. He took a train and a couple in the same compartment pointed out a house to him. Then he was with a woman, but knew she had a relationship with someone else. L's associations to the dream were somewhat hard to follow. The house seemed to remind him of some good memories of his childhood while staying with family friends when he arrived in this country. Apparently, his parents did not have sufficient space for him to live with them. I suggested his dream was about some of the losses in his life and what he missed. In response he repeated a story he'd told me about when, as a young man in some smart clothes, he'd been photographed by a fashion photographer. The photographer had given him his card, but as L was showing the card to someone, it blew out of his hand and was lost. He never saw the photographs. I said I felt he was sad about losing a good picture of himself, and good opportunities in his life. He replied by asking me how long it took for cyanide to kill you. He said someone once gave him a drink in a club. He thought it may have had cyanide in it. I think L experienced my interpretation about his sad feelings as something dangerous, even deadly.

For patients suffering from psychosis and violence, mourning may bring terrors of annihilation because it threatens the protective shield of the psychotic organization, which attempts to bind a fragile self together. The work of mourning involves achieving separateness through retrieving lost parts of the self, which in phantasy have been projected into members of the close knit gang of the organisation. Unravelling the projective processes would likely bring dread of fragmentation or unintegration. Mourning also means facing what may feel unbearable depressive feelings of remorse and sorrow about violence, feelings from which the psychotic organisation is a retreat.

As I indicated in the Introduction, I see the central importance to working through in therapy to enable the patient to retrieve projected parts of the self, and to mourn separateness and thereby gain a sense of having an integrated, autonomous identity (Steiner 1989). During the two years I spent in the unit I was unable to engage patients in ongoing therapy. The experiences which I have described with S and L were typical: patients usually dropped out after a few sessions. In part I think this was because of a lack of a safe, containing environment in this unit, an example of which was the denial of violence in the kind of lock on the door of the room used for therapy; and in part I think difficulties in my denial of violence, doubtless linked to difficulties in acknowledging my own hostility (Sedlak, 2019), also contributed. I decided to leave the unit because I felt too unsafe.

References

Bick, E. (1988 [1968]). The experience of the skin in early object relations. In E. Bott-Spillius (Ed.) *Melanie Klein To-day*, Vol. 1 (London: Routledge, 187–91).

Brownescombe Heller, M. (2003). Containment and counter-transference issues in a violent borderline patient. In R. Doctor (Ed.) *Dangerous Patients* (London: Karnac).

Campbell, D. and Hale, R. (1991). Suicidal acts. In J. Holmes (Ed.) *Textbook of Psychotherapy in Psychiatric Practice* (London: Churchill Livingstone, 287–306).

Caper, R. (1999). *A Mind of One's Own* (London: Routledge).

Fisher, J. and Ruszczynski, S. (1995). *Intimacy and the Couple.* London: Karnac.

Fonagy, P. and Target, M. (1999). Towards understanding violence: the use of the body and the role of the father. In R. Jozef Pereleberg (Ed.) *Psychoanalytic Understanding of Violence and Suicide* (London: Brunner Routledge).

Hyatt Williams, A. (1998). *Cruelty, Violence and Murder* (London: Karnac).

Klein. M. (1940). Mourning and its relation to manic-depressive states. *International Journal of Psychoanalysis, 21,* 125–153.

Klein, M. (1975 [1946]). Notes on some schizoid mechanisms. In *The Writings of Melanie Klein*, Vol. III (London: Hogarth, 1–24).

Pereleberg, R. J. (1999). Introduction. In R. Jozef Pereleberg (Ed.) *Psychoanalytic Understanding of Violence and Suicide* (London: Brunner Routledge).

Sedlak, V. (2019). *The Psychoanalyst's Superegos, Ego Ideals and Blind Spots: The Emotional Development of the Clinician.* London Routledge.

Steiner, J. (1989). The aim of psychoanalysis. *Psychoanalytic Psychotherapy*, 4, 109–20.

Steiner, J. (1993). *Psychic Retreats* (London: Routledge).

Chapter 5

Grief and Psychosis – The First Year of Therapy with J

Introduction

Although psychotherapy with people suffering from psychoses has become rare in public health settings, some years ago whilst taking up a newly established post as a psychotherapist in an acute psychiatric unit, I was able to engage in a four year, once weekly therapy with J, a man suffering from psychoses. I shall discuss the first year of the therapy in this chapter, and each of the following years in the next three chapters. In the discussion I include relevant psychoanalytic references. For readers unfamiliar with psychoanalytic literature about therapeutic work with people suffering from psychoses, please see Appendix 2. In Appendix 2 there is a summary of the main literature to which, in addition to weekly supervision, I turned for containment and support during the therapy with J.

In joining the psychiatric unit I found a welcome and interest in my psychodynamic approach, though the welcome was not without ambivalence. Quite literally the organisation took some time to make space for me. No room had been allocated for individual therapy. I was based in a rehabilitation unit with occupational therapists, working with in-patients and out-patients. For nine months I shared an open plan office. I had to book the large group meeting room to use for individual consultations. Then as a result of becoming acquainted with the nature of my work, and in a spirit of generosity which touched me, my new colleagues re-arranged their limited space to provide me with a separate office. This meant two staff had to move from their office into an even more cramped space which they shared with several others.

As I attended ward rounds, I saw and heard about the devastating effects of psychotic illnesses. My early impressions were of much grief. I encountered young people who seemed sentenced to spend the rest of their lives imprinted with a psychiatric diagnosis, dependent on a disability allowance. There were people in mid or late life returning to hospital with histories of multiple admissions, and lives littered with the wreckage of relationships, lives laid to waste. I thought the older patients were frightening messengers to the younger ones about what may lie ahead; and messengers to myself and other

DOI: 10.4324/9781003319719-9

staff about the destructiveness of a psychotic part of the mind. Much of the time the grief went unacknowledged by staff or patients.

Staff frequently complained about patients who lacked insight, meaning patients who denied they had a mental illness and failed to comply with their medication. I thought some of the difficulty in acknowledging a psychotic illness was the pain in grieving the damage that had been wrought by it, and mourning the hopes and dreams of the pre-damaged self. When I was asked to give a talk for the staff, I decided to speak about grief which accompanies a psychosis, and ordinary sadness as distinct from clinical depression. I discussed the need for opportunities to mourn the accompanying losses. In the talk I drew upon my experience of grief in working with old people who had suffered damaging physical illnesses like strokes (Terry, 2008).

I was shocked by how heavily medicated some of the patients were as they drifted around the wards like zombies. It seemed a cruel irony that many of these people, who came from a street drug culture, in hospital were obliged to give up their drugs for other drugs which often brought disabling and disturbing side effects. I thought they were also grieving the loss of their street drug induced highs when they felt more alive. I became aware of a drug dependent culture in the hospital evident in the frequent drug company sponsored lunches. A medical colleague admitted he felt guilty if he did not prescribe medication, and frightened that if he were summoned to court the first question would be about what medication he prescribed.

I found only a few referrals from the acute unit led to ongoing, out-patient therapy. During their stay in hospital many of those referred showed an openness and interest in exploring their emotional life. This seemed a testimony to the physical containment and safety provided by the hospital. However, once discharged, patients often returned in a closed up state, and seemed to feel it was too unsafe to continue any exploration of their feelings. For example some would say 'I don't want to talk about anything negative'. Regrettably there was an absence of residential units or day centres to which patients could be referred for psychotherapy. With some of those who continued in therapy I decided not to work interpretatively because they seemed too fragile. Instead I silently monitored the transference and counter-transference. With others, whom I felt were more robust, I explored an interpretative approach. This was not a hard and fast division, and sometimes I changed my mind, one way or the other.

A woman in her early twenties who attended for a just a few sessions seemed weighed down by medication. There were often long silences in which she struggled to think. On one such occasion I asked her about her silence. I felt encouraged by her reply that she was trying to remember her dreams. In a later session she was able to recall a dream in which she was holding a baby whom she thought was her own. She was upset because she noticed that the baby was disfigured on one side of its face. As we explored the dream, she became distressed after I suggested the baby might be. herself. I thought the dream was a painful evocation of the damaging effects of psychosis, as well as worries about passing on the psychosis to her offspring. Klein (1960, 1963) understood that people suffering from schizophrenia are vulnerable to guilt and depression, as a result of feeling responsible for splitting and destruction of something good in themselves and their good internal objects. This young woman had few memories of her childhood except an image of when she was little, lying on a bare table with a bright light above her. I thought this was a 'screen memory' (Freud, 1899) indicative of the lack of a holding maternal figure or primary carer. I did not make an interpretation about this memory. As this woman became more curious about herself, she told me she had spoken to her mother who told her to tell me she had often been in hospital for depression throughout her daughter's childhood. Perhaps fearfully anticipating or enacting her lack of early holding she soon dropped out of therapy.

The First Year with J

J was a man in his forties and an Asian immigrant. His father suffered from a psychotic illness, and J's mother went out to work. Later in J's life his father committed suicide. J suffered a breakdown in his adolescence and was hospitalized for several months. Afterwards he worked in a variety of jobs for some years before I saw him. He then suffered four breakdowns over a period of three years. In the breakdowns he experienced delusions and thought disorder. He was often in a suicidal state, and kept for a while in isolation under close watch. He had been diagnosed as suffering from schizophrenia. During his recovery from the fourth breakdown he was referred to me for psychotherapy. His diagnosis then was that he was suffering from a bi-polar disorder. He was prescribed lithium and anti-psychotic medication. For several months the work felt arid and stuck. Sometimes small movements would be followed by threats to discontinue the therapy. I discuss some of this fluctuation, the interactions between us which led to some development, and give an account of a session which brought a breakthrough.

J spoke English fluently but with an accent which for a while I found hard to understand. When I first saw him as an in-patient he was quite labile. He cried a great deal, particularly in relation to his father's suicide and his fear that he would follow in his father's footsteps. As he neared being discharged, he seemed to shore up his defences. He became rather silent and withdrawn. He complained about the therapy as though it was being imposed on him. The sullen withdrawal continued after he started attending as an out-patient. I began to feel whatever I said was of no use to him. He seemed to greet my efforts with a thinly veiled contempt. I am white and middle class. I found myself preoccupied with the cultural and racial differences between us. I ventured an interpretation saying I thought he felt I would never be able to understand his experience because of our different cultural and racial backgrounds. He then spoke more spontaneously, and described his experience of white people feeling superior to people of his race, who should work like dogs and have no time for talking. He said even within his own culture those who were wealthy looked down on poor people. My interpretation drew upon counter-transference feelings of helplessness and inadequacy, and my struggle to understand J. The interpretation brought some contact with J when he felt I understood his despair about me. He revealed a view of me in the transference as someone who felt superior to him, thought he should be working like a dog and should not be engaged in a talking therapy. I thought these views probably reflected his experiences of racism which were internalised in a superior psychotic part of his mind, which was opposed to the sane part of his mind's therapeutic alliance with me.

The contact between us improved a little, but he again brought worries about whether he might commit suicide. He came to a session saying he felt suicidal, it was too much of a struggle. It would be better to end it all. Later in this session, he brought a dream in which he witnessed a man murdering a woman. J became frightened he too would be murdered and ran away. When I took this up in the transference, in terms of his fears of me and the struggle to come and talk to me, he agreed. He said he has buried things all these years. He felt frightened to look at the darker side of himself and of what might emerge from the therapy. I pointed out to him that though he said the murder in the dream took place in the dark, he was a witness. I said I felt this indicated a part of him who, despite his fears, wanted to bring his thoughts and dreams so we could understand them. I also spoke of a murderous part which hated feelings and his interest in his emotional life, and wanted to kill off any contact between us. After this session I was left feeling worried about J's suicidal thoughts. I later spoke to his key worker about my concerns.

I think the improving contact led to a negative therapeutic reaction expressed in J's suicidal feelings. These feelings were an attack on the developing relationship from a psychotic part of his mind, revealed in his dream as a murderous and frightening figure. J was frightened about what was emerging in the dream from his unconscious. In my interpretations I aimed to support and distinguish the sane part of his mind, his ego which was allied with me in therapy. Although frightened, he was observing a murderous psychotic part and bringing observations in the form of the dream to therapy. His fears were projectively evoked in me, and I worried about his potential suicidality.

The improved contact with J continued only for a short while. He subsequently became withdrawn and rather recalcitrant. He complained of a lack of interest in anything. In one session he spoke nostalgically about his former interest in walking in the country. He told me in the countryside he liked to go slowly, not to frighten the animals, to meditate and breathe deeply. Robert Langs (1978) has drawn attention to how our patients sometimes offer us supervision. I took the country walking story as advice about how I should proceed.

The following sessions again felt stuck. There was little sense of movement, except I felt J seemed to value a meditative quality of some of the silences. However, I heard that when he met his registrar for the routine monitoring of his medication, he made jokes about the two of us sitting in silence. He began to arrive late for his sessions. On one occasion he came late saying he felt he had benefitted enough from the therapy, or perhaps he was unable to benefit any more. When I took up his lateness, he said my clock must be fast. I replied I thought it was nonsense to say he had benefitted enough because he brought the same complaints; but I thought there was a tricky part of him which tried to persuade him my clock was too fast and that he couldn't benefit from psychotherapy. At the next session he was not so late. He talked of a part time job he'd seen which involved unpacking frozen meat. He couldn't bring himself to apply for it. I spoke about his interest in and reluctance about unpacking his feelings, which have been frozen for a long time. He agreed and said perhaps it was better left frozen. He then told me he had some dreams but couldn't recall them. I said perhaps he could write them down.

The meditative quality of the silences seemed in the spirit of the supervisory advice J had offered about going slowly. But the superior, psychotic part of J's mind ridiculed the silences. It attempted to undermine the therapy in his jokes with the registrar, and doubtless influenced his repeated lateness. When I challenged the sane part of his mind to see the falseness in this propaganda, he could bring his sane part's fears about unpacking his frozen emotions. Interpreting those fears led to a bit of unfreezing when he mentioned dreams he couldn't recall. My suggestion to write down his dreams was again to support his ego or the sane part of his mind, which was interested in unpacking his dreams.

He came early the following week and described four dreams. Two of these dreams were about stray dogs, and one about a favourite teacher who was teaching him a new subject. I understood the dreams as poignant indications of his stray dog self and a developing positive transference. For the next three months he continued to bring at least three or four dreams to each session. There were recurring images which I thought were transparent references to his breakdowns: bicycles with broken wheels, cars or buses breaking down. The threatening male figure reappeared whom either J witnessed killing someone or who was known to be a murderer. J would recount all the dreams at once. He would fall silent waiting for me to talk about the dreams. My supervisor and I puzzled over this process. I decided not to try to interpret it to him, but simply to follow his country walking advice and wait. Following a break he again came complaining, saying he couldn't understand why I insisted he attend therapy. I hadn't insisted he attend but his repeated complaints that I did reflected a projection of his sane part's recognition of his need of the therapy, despite the opposition of the psychotic part.

Two weeks later there was a breakthrough in a session in which J arrived and reported the following dreams:

He is bicycling with a friend and they both get flat tyres on the front wheels. They leave the bikes at a bus station and catch a bus.

In the second dream he is watering his garden, a friend or neighbour is also watering a garden. J sees a snake and it bites him. The neighbour sees an even bigger snake and manages to catch it.

In the third dream he asks a friend to go to the Rehab with him. The friend laughs sarcastically. This friend doesn't know about J's mental disability. The friend says he would have to lose his head to go to Rehab.

Having told the dreams, J pauses and waits. I say perhaps he feels flat like the tyres. He looks at me and agrees. He says that's just how he feels, slowed down. He is silent again. I say it is difficult for him to bring his more vulnerable feelings, like flatness or upset feelings. There seems to be a part of him, shown in the Rehab dream, who pours scorn on the therapy. Sensing he may not have understood my use of 'scorn', I ask him if he understands what I meant. He says no he doesn't understand. I talk about looking down one's nose at something, and he nods.

After a few minutes silence, he talks of a dog which got into his flat, and his struggle to catch it and get rid of it. He says it scared the shit out of him. He goes on to say that he feels frightened about his illness, that he won't recover as before. He says it's a big effort to do anything. He feels he is dragging himself through the day. It is much harder when there's nothing to do. He says there's a limit to how much TV you can watch. He limits himself to two or three hours a day. It's good when he can find something interesting to read, that helps him sleep. I ask if he has found something to read. He laughs saying he thinks of going to the library, but he keeps procrastinating. He says sometimes he phones a help line several times a day for a chat. He hasn't phoned recently because he thinks the girls he speaks to are getting fed up with him. J talks about this in a matter of fact, stoical way, but I feel shocked.

He says he doesn't want to keep mixing with people who also have a disability like him. He asks 'Who can you meet during the day when most people are at work?' He has made a friend of a taxi driver whom he sees at weekends. The taxi driver smokes pot, is often in a dreamy state and speaking in a way that doesn't make much sense. I say perhaps he worries about talking to me that I will get fed up with him like the help line girls; or that I am like this dreamy taxi driver only interested in his dreams and speaking in a way which doesn't make sense. He replies, speaking with determination, that he will talk about anything if asked. Otherwise he will talk when he's in the mood and ready to do so.

J readily agreed to my interpretation about his flat feelings like the flat tyres, but then seemed to withdraw again. I think the flatness was despair about the therapy promoted by a sarcastic psychotic part, allegedly a friend, who denigrates the therapy and denies the psychosis or 'disability'. In contrast, a sane part in the dream knows about his disability and is engaged in the rehab therapy with me. The interpretation of the denigration by the psychotic part, led to his association about the dog in his flat, which indicated how frightened he was of the psychotic part. He then seemed less intimidated by the psychotic part. For the first time he revealed details of his daily life, the desperation and emptiness he felt.

Concluding Reflections on the First Year

I understand J's oscillation in and out of emotional contact as his tentative ventures from a psychotic organisation in the mind (Steiner, 1993). The organisation offered him a refuge from the fears of breaking down again and the dread of unintegration or fragmentation. The psychotic organisation was also a retreat from the pain of depressive feelings. A number of the dreams emerging in this first year included images resonant with the damage wrought by psychosis. The acknowledgment in the dreams of the damage brings the possibility of mourning, with the painful internal work of sorting out what can be salvaged and what is irretrievably lost. The therapeutic task is similar to the working through for people suffering the aftermath of post-traumatic stress disorder (Garland, 1998). People who have experienced psychotic breakdowns are survivors of an internal catastrophe, a destruction of their minds. Like the survivors of external disasters, they face the task of mourning the loss of their pre-trauma self, and the recognition that they can never return to that former state. The worry accompanying the working through in mourning is that the pain of depressive feelings of sadness, sorrow and remorse might propel these patients back into a psychotic state. Valerie Sinason (1992) has discussed how people suffering from intellectual disability also need to mourn considerable damage, but they can feel it better to be mad rather than sad.

The development in the work with J was somewhat in reverse to some expectations in therapy. Usually there is a hope dreams will eventually emerge as a result of developing capacities to symbolize and metabolize experience. Instead, I felt swamped by dream material. I struggled to remember all the dreams that were introduced at the beginning of each session. It was such an enormous step for J to bring this dream material that I was hesitant to address the way in which he brought the dreams. He seemed to wait for me to comment like some kind of oracle. I found I needed to wait and try to make something of the dreams, thinking of the several dreams almost as one continuous dream.

J continued to bring more of his life, the bleakness was upsetting to hear. It was painful too as he tried to make sense of the psychosis and its implications for the present and future. For much of the time I felt J's sense of his capacities were projectively located in me, because of the pain which would come from him being in touch both with his damage as well as his capacities. He looked to me to see what I understood were his capacities. For example, having already signed up for jury service, he asked if I thought he could do it. After he was accepted for the jury service he again brought various worries about his ability to take part. He became reassured when he had the thought there would be others with him on the jury trying to reach a decision together. He said he was struck by how important the jury were, they came in last, after the judge, and seemed even more important than the judge. I thought J was then less in a frozen state. He was in touch with more resources, an internal world with more helpful figures, not so frightened or dominated by a psychotic part.

Later, just before a break, he brought a dream in which he was beginning to stand up to the sarcasm of the psychotic part. In the same session he mentioned a review tribunal he had to attend each year in which he would be asked whether he thought he was someone with a mental illness. He felt very perplexed by what answer to give. He worried that if he said he didn't think he was ill he might be charged for an incident which occurred before he was hospitalised. He believed the charge against him was unjust. At the time it was easier to be let off the charge because of his illness, than to contest it. J was beginning to explore how his sane part could be compromised by a collusive liaison with the psychotic part. In view of the imminent break, and the anticipation of depressive feelings connected with the loss of the therapeutic relationship, he was particularly vulnerable to such a collusion to escape the pain of loss. Following the break, on the day of my return to the unit, J was admitted in a psychotic state. He was not able to manage the depressive feelings stirred in my absence. He recovered enough to be discharged quite quickly, and the therapy continued. He talked for the first time about being troubled by his intense involvement in sex in frequent visits to 'sex workers'. He had been going to sex workers since his late adolescence, but his visits increased following his first breakdown. Despite his still somewhat agitated, manic state there was some calm. J and I could think about a link between this use of sex and a need to lift himself over painful depressive feelings.

References

Freud, S. (1899). Screen Memories, S.E. 3.

Garland, C. (1998). *Understanding Trauma*. London: Duckworth.

Klein, M. (1960). Symposium on 'Depressive Illness' – V. a Note on Depression in the Schizophrenic. *International Journal of Psychoanalysis, 41,* 509–11.

Langs, R. (1978). *The Listening Process*. New York: Aronson.

Sinason, V. (1992). *Mental Handicap and The Human Condition*. London: Free Association.

Steiner, J. (1993). *Psychic Retreats*. London: Routledge.

Terry, P. (2008). *Counselling and Psychotherapy with Older People: A Psychodynamic Approach*. London: Palgrave Macmillan.

Chapter 6

Encounters with a Psychotic Superego – The Second Year of Therapy with J

Introduction

A few months into the second year of the therapy I offered to present some clinical material to a small, ad hoc group of therapist colleagues. The group was specially convened for a one-off opportunity for supervision by a psychoanalyst who was visiting the area in which we worked. It was the first time I had presented before these colleagues. I read a process recording of a verbatim account made from memory of the dialogue of a recent session with J. After I finished reading the process recording there was an awkward silence. The visiting analyst turned to me and, with barely concealed impatience, said, 'You've avoided the transference!' Worse followed. My colleagues tried in vain to offer support. I felt numbed, in a state of shock because, whilst I could just about see what was being pointed out, otherwise I could hardly think. More shocking to me, and something I could scarcely admit to myself, was that prior to the supervision I thought it was good work. Dare I admit it, as I went into the supervision group, I remember thinking 'Well, what will there be to discuss!' This alarming omnipotence was punctured by the visiting analyst. I felt paralysed by the analyst's comments which I experienced as condemnations from an omniscient, psychoanalytic superego. Later, I understood the supervision experience enacted a 'parallel process' of the therapy which Mattison (1975) describes can occur when dynamics of the therapist and patient relationship are reflected in a supervisory relationship. In this instance I believe the parallel process was one in which I was enacting my experience with J. Unconsciously I was letting the supervisor know something of what it was like for me to be with J when he seemed in thrall to a psychotic superego.

Harold Searles (1979) in his book on counter-transference, writing with disarming candour about therapy which had extended over 18 years with a woman suffering from psychosis, wrote:

> 'I had the thought that I have been having my psychoses vicariously in a controlled way through her, over the years, with my being safely apart

DOI: 10.4324/9781003319719-10

from it, and that the hundreds of tapes of our sessions in my storeroom represent this psychosis of mine'.

(Searles 1979, p. 418)

He describes an experience of vulnerability and omnipotence which echoed my experience. He wrote about his training analysis saying:

'On the one hand, I was convinced that I was on the verge of such overwhelming insanity that I frequently admonished the analyst "You'd better get a bed ready for me at Chestnut Lodge" – the very hospital in which Searles ended up treating his psychotic patients. He continued: 'On the other hand, I was convinced that I was so manifestly and totally well that the analysis had now become absurdly superfluous'.

(Searles 1979, p. 480–1)

Late in her career Klein made references to 'terrifying figures' in deep layers of the unconscious, which remain unmodified by experience and development (Klein 1958, p. 241–3). Rosenfeld (1952) described 'a particularly severe superego of a persecutory nature' in people suffering from schizophrenia. He suggested that modifications in analytic technique, such as reassurance and control, which were introduced into the early psychoanalytic treatments, were responses to the terrifying nature of the superego in schizophrenia. The modifications, particularly the reluctance to address negative aspects of the transference, can be understood as counter-transference enactments out of fear of the patient's superego.

Albert Mason (1981) indicated how a 'suffocating superego' can lead to psychosis. Writing in tribute to the influence that Bion had on his work with psychotic patients, Mason describes a suffocating superego which he contrasts with a normal superego or conscience. It is particularly the quality of omnipotence to which he draws attention, an implacable omnipotence born of the 'implacable fantasies of the helpless infant', whose 'only weapon against terrifying helplessness is his mind and organs of perception' used in fantasy to control and possess the primary maternal figure. Mason writes: 'This nipple possessed and surrounded by the child's mouth, trapped and controlled, in fact virtually devoured, will later, when introjected into the ego, become a superego component which will be felt to surround, trap, devour and suffocate the child's personality in fantasy, producing the internal claustrophobia and acute psychotic breaks' (Mason 1981, p. 145). Mason vividly describes how this suffocating superego creates 'a sensation in the mind of being watched by eyes from which nothing can escape. These eyes are cruel, penetrating, inhuman and untiring. They record without mercy, pity or compassion. They follow relentlessly and judge remorselessly. No escape is possible for there is no place to shelter. Their memory is infinite and their threat is nameless. The punishment when it comes will be swift, poisonous and ruthless ... Added to this feeling of being constantly watched and threatened there is also the sense of being acutely listened to, smelled and even having one's thoughts read'. Mason explains that the resulting feelings of hopelessness and terror are caused not only 'because of a belief engendered that no escape is possible, but the crushing and suffocating quality also produces panic and explosion, in a desperate attempt to escape, even at the cost of disintegration' (Mason 1981, p. 143). De Masi (2001) describes a 'psychotic superego' as 'full of terrorizing objects', which he says 'cannot be compared with the neurotic superego which stems from the introjection of parental figures, albeit with degrees of distortion' (2001, p. 90). A psychotic superego can terrorise therapists, hijack their minds and hold their clinical acumen to ransom.

The Second Year

As a result of reviewing the session which I took to the group supervision several themes stood out. The themes had arisen in some previous sessions and J had returned to them, a likely indication I had not understood them. The themes had transference implications which, as the visiting analyst noted, I failed to address. J had spoken again of worrying about being unable to stop going to the sex workers, and the large sums of money he spent seeing them. He could ill afford it and worried how it depleted his limited resources. A second more recent theme was about his efforts to resume some part time work as a hairdresser. He said his clients tell him all sorts of stories, 'it's therapy'. He talked about advertising for doing hair dressing in clients' homes, but he worried about gay clients who expect sexual favours. A third theme was about his loneliness, his wish to have a child, and his thinking about advertising for a surrogate mother. With the benefit of hindsight the aspects of the transference in these themes, which I see were missed, are an ambivalent mix of feelings about his need of me. On the one hand there was a denial of his need of me. I was condemned as a sex worker who exploits him and drains his resources; or condemned as a gay hairdressing client who wants sexual favours from him, and for whom J provides therapy. On the other hand J's wished for a child contains his projected infantile need for myself as a surrogate mother therapist.

The week after my experience in the supervision group, J came with news that he was joining a voluntary euthanasia group. He explained that looking ahead to when his mother dies, euthanasia would be a solution from his mental torture. When I took up his sense of hopelessness about relying on me to help him, I felt sharply rebuked when he replied he must rely on himself, that's all he can rely on. In the following session he reiterated his plans for euthanasia, having now located a doctor who would help him. Again he dismissed any suggestion he might need me. It seemed it would be better to be dead than depend on me. I struggled to think, reeling from his plan about euthanasia, and from an inner condemnation of myself in the aftermath of the supervision group.

In the next few weeks J talked about the Olympic games which were then taking place. He brought some dreams which had an atmosphere of winning and confidence, signalling some emerging feeling of hopefulness. But there were also developments in the euthanasia project. The doctor, whom J had found, was marketing a death kit. When I interpreted a longing to win a special Olympic prize place with me J looked puzzled. He said he couldn't see how he would want to be special to me. He went on to tell me about the incompetent tutors who were teaching the 'back to work' course he was attending, confirming in the transference his poor view of me. J came to the next session saying that he'd been thinking about his going to the sex workers, he'd been analysing himself. He thought he must be going to the sex workers to cover over his real self, like a mask. I wondered about an omnipotence in his reference to analysing himself, but decided to simply acknowledge his reflectiveness. He went on to explain that when he sees the girls who are using heroin and other abusive substances, he feels better off. He repeated various worries: about the money he spends on the girls, his frustration about not having a job which drives him to them, his fears of having another breakdown if he were to work again, and wondering whether he should risk it anyway.

As this session proceeded, I again found myself struggling to think. Gradually I recovered and made some interpretations about his worries during the rest of the session. I said I think he is drawn to going to the sex workers because he can feel that his needy self is in them, and then his needy self gets covered over. His need for me is frustrated with just a brief contact of once a week, and perhaps he feels I don't understand just how frustrating it is. But when he is with the sex workers, he feels the needs are in them, and that they are in trouble because of their needs. Ordinary needs to be known and understood get mixed up with destructiveness which drains his resources. When he is frightened of breaking down again, he especially needs to be held and understood. J seemed to ignore the interpretations, but later mentioned wanting to be touched when he is with the sex workers. He added sadly that it isn't the same with a stranger. Somewhat later referring to the two of us, he said he sees it as just two minds meeting to try to think about his problems. I replied that he leaves out any feelings, whereas I think when he feels I understand him he feels touched, and this is very important to him. I felt this session was something of a breakthrough because I was able to recover some capacity to think.

The next week J complained of feeling like a zombie and of needing to be in hospital. He had even asked his doctor to give him ECT (electroconvulsive therapy). He said he was trying to keep occupied. He cleaned one of his bedroom windows. It took him twice as long as it should have and he felt exhausted. I thought the previous week had given us a clearer view, but he found it too painful to continue looking. J was in much the same state the following week, insisting there was no change. He introduced a theme which was to preoccupy him over the following weeks: he became increasingly impelled to find a means of identifying anonymous telephone callers who would not reveal their phone numbers. He was angry that it was the callers whose privacy was protected because they could choose whether to identify themselves or not. Whereas he thought those who received the calls should be protected. My supervisor, a psychoanalyst whom I consulted individually each week, drew my attention to J's need to protect himself. Perhaps he was the recipient of invasive projections as an infant or perhaps some abuse.

The next week J was much more upset about identifying anonymous callers. He was spending a lot of time writing letters of complaint. He worried that he was breaking down again. I wondered how it was that he was receiving so many calls. It emerged that he had started advertising for hairdressing work. He described some of the calls responding to his ads as disturbing, like being emotionally molested. I found listening to him disturbing. Rather atypically I started making interpretations of an historical kind, repeatedly trying to link J's current concerns with speculations about his past. He did his best to ignore these interpretations. Only in supervision did I realise the session had turned into an enactment of me trying to force an understanding of the causes of his disturbance into him. The next week was even more unsettling. J came saying he felt he was getting a bit high. He was more and more agitated about the telephone calls. There were calls disturbing him from gay men and telemarketing companies asking strange questions, which he felt were up to some sort of monkey business. He was recording the licence numbers of cars and other vehicles which overtook him, or intruded into his lane when he was driving. I felt unable to think. Only later in supervision did I appreciate just how frightened and helpless I felt and how my experience gave some clues to J's feelings.

The following session J did not turn up for his appointment, the first time he had missed a session. I wanted to phone him but struggled with this because of all the material about the telephone calls. I worried phoning might be a further enactment of my intruding into him. As his session time elapsed, in the last ten minutes I decided to phone. He answered but seemed dazed and confused. He spoke of extra medication he was recently prescribed. I offered him a later session on the same day. He came to this session saying he'd forgotten the appointment. I said it wasn't like him. He talked about the extra medication which made him sleep longer. He had decided to stop taking it. He went on to say he had received a phone bill which omitted some charges. He wondered whether this was to keep him happy in view of the complaints he'd made. He talked of his continuing preoccupation with finding a phone which could block anonymous calls. Then, more thoughtfully he said he didn't know why these minutiae are so important to him, though it was satisfying trying to get it right.

I replied I thought his preoccupation with the phones and trying to block callers who won't identify themselves, was linked with something that we had identified in our work together and which he was now trying to block from awareness. We had seen how his need to be held and understood by me was covered over by going to the sex workers, whom he felt were needy and in trouble. These needs were frightening and painful, which was why they had to be blocked from awareness. After being silent for a little while he said he hasn't been going to the sex workers so much recently. He was too busy with his concerns about the phones, and it is good he hasn't gone to them. I said he saw some benefits in these preoccupations about the phones. Perhaps he blocked taking in what I was showing him. After more silence he talked of wanting to have a child, and wanting to donate sperm.

J came back the next week saying that he had seen an advertisement for a course about writing an autobiography. He had a dream in which someone was telling him to do the course. He spoke sadly of having forgotten a lot of things about his life because of the medication or ECT. He had listened to messages he had left on answerphones when he was ill, but he had no memory of them now. Later, he said he had bought a new toy, some software, which he had been trying with some difficulty to install by himself. It would give him access to e-mail and the internet. He described some excitement about the possibilities. He'd been so involved that he hadn't been going to the sex workers. Again I noticed but did not refer to the possible omnipotence in the reference to installing the software by himself. I said that feeling more in touch with a boy inside him who needs me, wants to be here and play, opens up all sorts of possibilities for discovering more about himself and his capacities. J returned to worries about going back to the sex workers, about his illness, not being able to work again, and worries about his preoccupations with the phones and telephone salesmen. When I interpreted the worries as taking him away from thinking about the boy within him, he was silent for a while. I asked him what he was thinking. He said he was thinking about what I said about the boy. He turned to me and asked 'Why am I frightened of the boy?' I said that is a good question. I think it's frightening to be aware of the intensity of the boy's needs, his passionate feelings and need of me. J went on to talk of his enthusiasm about e-mail because whoever writes to you, their address can be identified. I said I thought he wasn't frightened of the boy at that moment. He could identify where his feelings were coming from, and that opened up all kinds of opportunities.

We were now approaching a second Christmas holiday. In the next week's session J continued to speak enthusiastically about the various possibilities of the internet, particularly the value of being able to converse with others. He recalled a woman who had helped him when he had been ill. When I suggested he felt that his conversations with me were helping, he replied 'Well yes, any conversation helps even if it is fruitless'. The following week J began by saying that he was going to place an advertisement in some papers for a surrogate mother. The advertisement would read: 'Wanted a compassionate surrogate mother'. He said he had first thought of being a donor to the IVF programme to help a childless couple have a baby, but when he obtained the application forms he realised he wouldn't be accepted. So the next plan was to have a child of his own, which would make him more like normal people and it easier to find a partner. I said I thought his feelings, about wanting a child and to be normal like others, were mixed with feeling rejected when I leave him. He felt I was part of a couple going away and leaving him. A little fellow inside him wanted a compassionate mother to look after him, not a mother therapist who goes away and leaves him. J then spoke of his registrar whom he liked and felt took an interest in him. She was leaving the hospital at Christmas. But, he said, he told himself, as he told others, that we all have twins. When someone goes an even better twin will come along. I said I thought there was twin J who was telling the sad and unhappy twin who misses me, and the doctor, not to mind, to look on the bright side. Someone else will come, someone even better to replace me. J looked pleasantly surprised. He said, 'I've always been looking on the bright side all my life. There are some things you just can't control and you have to accept. Feeling sad can drive you crazy if you go on being sad all the time'. I said I felt J was frightened of sad, out of control feelings, afraid perhaps of being suicidal like his father. Later, after a silence I asked J what he was thinking. He replied that he was thinking about these things he'd not thought of before. He said he didn't seem to have any feelings, and perhaps that's why he'd lost lots of friends. I said I thought it wasn't that he didn't have feelings, but that he wasn't able to be aware of them. There was probably too much out of control going on, but I thought he was aware of his feelings now. Painful feelings about losing a friendly me who showed him things he hadn't thought before.

Concluding Reflections on the Second Year

After I presented at the group supervision with the visiting analyst, I was shocked by the omnipotence which had consumed me in the way I thought about the work I was to present and in the way I heard the criticism of it. I felt spoken to as though I had no understanding of transference, almost as though I'd never heard of it. Still a newcomer to the group I worried that whatever reputation I had would soon, once word got around, be in tatters. I might as well throw in the sponge, hand in the towel, call it a day, give up. In the subsequent therapy with J I felt alarmed by his plans for euthanasia, his request for ECT, and his disturbance about the unidentified phone calls which he seemed to be attracting in his advertisements for work. My supervisor helped me to reflect on my overwhelming feelings of being frightened and helpless, and see they were a communication about J's feelings. I came to understand more clearly that J's retreat to a psychotic organisation included an omnipotent psychotic superego which ruthlessly attacked any helpful link between us.

Joan Symington's thoughts about the survival aspects of omnipotence were important. Drawing on Bick's work, Symington (1985) notes that attacks on dependency in the therapeutic relationship derive from a primitive, muscular stiffening against an infantile dread of unintegration. Symington notes feelings of infantile dependency and helplessness can bring terrible reminders of being unheld, of 'spilling into space'. The hard ruthless attacks, my mental paralysis and J's self reported zombie like state, may be different aspects of this mental stiffening against a dread of unintegration, which were likely prompted by feeling unheld. When I struggled to think under relentless attacks from J's superego and from my own, I found it hard to hold onto any sense of my own capacities. I thus had a glimpse of the assaults by a psychotic part of the mind on the mind itself, and the ensuing despair and hopelessness.

Often J seemed to ignore what I said, and rarely looked at me. Perhaps I was to know something of his experience of being with an impermeable object, unable to contain or even register his emotional states; or perhaps this was another way of him stiffening himself against fears of unintegration. When J brought his plans for euthanasia, though I was alarmed I think it was important I could bear the terrible hopelessness. This containment led to a brief period of hopefulness where I felt we gained some understanding of a needy self which he lodged in the sex workers he visited. It seemed developments were often intertwined with omnipotence. As I tried to tease out different strands it was difficult to decide what to address. For example when he brought some thoughts about himself going to the sex workers whether to take up the omnipotence in his 'analysing' himself or his reflectiveness. I decided not to interpret the omnipotence. Rosenfeld (1987) described a 'thin skinned narcissism' which is associated with very traumatized patients. He thought that for such patients, interpretations of destructiveness can add to the trauma already experienced (Rosenfeld 1987, pp. 274–5). Joan Symington (1985) also warns about only interpreting destructiveness and not acknowledging the survival aspects of the omnipotent defences.

At times I felt I became not just an inadequate container, but also a leaky one, trying to force things into him, misinterpreting his advertisements, molesting him with interpretations. I tended to become so worried about being identified with an invasive and abusive telephone caller that when, unusually J failed to attend his session, it was enormously difficult to decide whether to phone him. It turned out phoning was alright. My supervisor later said: 'quite simple actions can speak volumes'. My supervisor, doubtless held my helpless, infantile self. She helped me find a means of speaking about and to an infant J, in a way that he could eventually hear and become curious about. As we approached the Christmas holiday, J acknowledged some of the interpretations about the boy. He could let me know that despite a psychotic superego's withering view of the fruitlessness of our conversations, he was thinking of things he'd not thought before.

References

Bick, E. (1968). The experience of skin in early object relations. In E. Bott-Spillius E. (Ed.) *Melanie Klein To-day, Volume 1*. London: Routledge.

De Masi, F. (2001). The unconscious and psychosis: some considerations of the psychoanalytic theory of psychosis. In P. Williams (Ed.) *Language for Psychosis.* London: Whurr.

Klein, M. (1958). On the development of mental functioning. *International Journal of Psychoanalysis, 39,* 84–90.

Mason, A. (1981). The suffocating superego: Psychotic breaks and claustrophobia. In J. Grotstein (Ed.) *Do I Dare Disturb the Universe?* London: Karnac.

Mattinson, J. (1975). *The Reflection Process in Casework Supervision.* London: Institute of Martial Studies, The Tavistock Institute of Human Relations.

Rosenfeld, H. (1952). Notes on the psychoanalysis of the superego conflict of an acute schizophrenic patient. *International Journal of Psychoanalysis, 33,* 111–31.

Rosenfeld, H. (1987). *Impasse and Interpretation.* London: Tavistock.

Searles, H.F. (1979). *Countertransference.* New York: International Universities Press.

Symington, J. (1985). The survival function of primitive omnipotence. *International Journal of Psychoanalysis 66,* 481–7.

Chapter 7

Struggles to Contain Madness – The Third Year of Therapy with J

Introduction

Robert Caper (1999) notes that Bion developed his seminal concept of containment from analysing people suffering from psychosis, in essence from containing psychotic aspects of emotional experience, which Bion described as 'beta elements'. Caper elucidates Bion's insight that containment can mean the therapist bearing experiences which are hardly states of mind at all and consist of:

> 'unconscious delusions, hallucinations, bizarre objects and moralistic hatred…concrete experiences that cannot be encompassed (borne) by the mind, i.e. thought about, doubted or tested, because they encompass, invade and deaden the mind instead'.
>
> (Caper, 1999, p.148)

In containment, Caper differentiates two different and often co-existing motives of projective identification: an 'urgent' need for someone else to bear the unbearable with the hope that it may eventually be transformed and retrieved; and an 'aggressive' motive to control the other person. In Bion's writings about containment Caper draws attention to a hitherto overlooked reference to the role of the father, which develops some aspects discussed in Chapter 4 about the role of the father or third figure. Bion wrote:

> 'if the feeding mother cannot allow reverie or if the reverie is allowed but is not associated with love for the child or its father this fact will be communicated to the infant even though incomprehensible to the infant'.
>
> (Bion quoted by Caper, 1999, p. 119)

It is Bion's inclusion of the importance of mother's love for the father which Caper notes as overlooked and puzzling. Caper explains this importance in the following way. Whilst the mother, or primary carer needs a capacity for receptiveness to the infant's projections, she also needs a passionate attachment to the father or some other third figure, to help her disentangle herself from the

DOI: 10.4324/9781003319719-11

infant's projections. For the mother and baby, what is important is father's or third figure's capacity to maintain some distance, to protect the boundaries around the nursing couple, and help mother and infant separate. Within the process of containment it can be useful to distinguish between a maternal receptiveness to the infant's projections, a paternal distance from them, and a link between the maternal and paternal capacities in which there can be some creative thought to process and transform the projections. Caper develops the therapeutic implications of this conceptualization by describing the import-ance of the therapist's love of psycho-analysis, meaning not an idealization or identification with psycho-analysis but a passionate attachment. This love establishes psycho-analysis as an internal paternal object which helps the therapist not be dominated by the patient's projections, or become merged with the patient in a maternal transference and counter-transference. Caper proposes it is the link between the capacity of the therapist to be receptive to the patient's projections, and the capacity to distance him or herself from them, that enables the therapist to become the good combined maternal-paternal object for the non-narcissistic part of the patient i.e. the part of the patient which hopes the projections can be transformed and returned, as dis-tinct from a narcissistic or psychotic part which uses the projections to control and maintain a state of merger.

The therapists' relationship in their minds with a third perspective is also vitally important in any therapy, but can be difficult to sustain. Caper discusses how therapists often become aware they have been taken over by the patient's projections in supervision. For example it is not uncommon for members of a group supervision to see an apparently obvious aspect of the therapeutic interaction to which the presenting therapist seemed blinded. As a result of containing aspects of the patient's experience, including the omnipotent phantasy in projective identification of being able to take over someone else's mind, the therapist's mind may temporarily join in this delu-sion until released by a third perspective of supervision. At other times the therapist makes this recovery either within a session or outside of it by linking up again with a relationship with an internal psychoanalytic object.

Caper's stress on the importance of a relationship in the mind with a third perspective has much in common with Britton's (1989) seminal work on tri-angular space for thinking. Britton discussed how this space is created in the mind following the recognition of the parental sexual relationship, a rec-ognition that goes hand-in-hand with the working through of the Oedipus complex and the depressive position. Britton draws attention to the way early difficulties in containment can make it dangerous to recognise the parental relationship. Failures in maternal containment can mean that in order to pre-serve a good life-giving mother, bad uncontaining and life threatening aspects of the mother are split off, externally into the father and internally into a destructive superego. A good mother is felt to be essential to life, and conse-quently a connection between a good mother and a bad father can be felt to be disastrous and life threatening. Britton (1989, p. 90) discusses how the result of this dilemma for someone suffering from psychosis can mean that to avoid a parental connection in the mind, the patient will in omnipotent phantasy destroy his or her mind. Hence, working therapeutically with people suffering from psychosis can present a tension for the therapist between holding a link with a third perspective in his or her mind in order to be able to think, and doing so in such a way that will not exacerbate the patient's psychotic state of mind.

The Third Year of Therapy

The year began with a shaky start. J returned after the Christmas break in an agitated state. He was particularly worried about difficulties in sleeping, convinced if he continued to lose sleep he would break down again. In the second week back, J came to his session in a state of shock saying he had crashed his car the previous day. He had taken a heavy dose of sleeping tablets which he obtained from a GP. The tablets didn't seem to have any effect. He went for a drive and fell asleep at the wheel. In the following weeks J seemed to crash from a manic state. He became in touch with a painful vulnerability. In his upset about the car he struggled with feelings, particularly his despair about his own sense of damage. For a while he continued trying to sort out what could be repaired of his life and what was irreparable.

J came to a session saying he was attempting to sell his flat in order to move away from a neighbour who was trying to take over his garden. He said the neighbour wanted to stop him trimming the garden. J said he likes to trim the garden, clearing the undergrowth is important to him. I said when he felt more hopeful about the work he and I were doing in clearing the undergrowth of his mind, then a part of him tries to pull him away, tries to persuade him I am trying to take over his mind and control him. J was silent. After a while he said sadly, 'That's what I do, often, when I think other people are trying to control me'. This was an arresting moment of contact. It was most unusual for J to pause, consider an interpretation in this way, tell me his thoughts and agree with what I had shown him.

The next week I crashed. I had a raging toothache and cancelled the session at short notice. I could not contact J but left a message for him on his answer machine, offering an alternative appointment later in the week. Although he received the message, he turned up at his usual session time. He was distraught. He told my colleagues he was finishing the therapy, and would not see me again. A few hours later he was admitted to the acute unit. When I next saw him, he was in the locked ward, heavily medicated with scared, bloodshot eyes. He insisted he didn't want to see me again, that he had pressed the delete button on the therapy. In a groggy voice I could barely decipher, he spoke with much anguish about police who had circled a man with a knife and shot him through the heart. (This incident had been reported in the news some time previously.) Sobbing, he told me he feared he would lose his disability pension because he was getting too well. He said it was his dream he would always have the disability pension, it was a comfort. Later, my supervisor discussed with me how my sudden cancellation of J's appointment had shot him through the heart, shot through his dream he and I would always be together, a shocking betrayal.

The following week he came from the ward to his session. He was tearful and seemed lost. He remained for a month on the ward, a long time by comparison with the usual practice in which it was rare for patients to stay for more than several days. J broke down three more times in the next five months. Throughout that time there was a relentless repetitiveness about the sessions. I would feel I was peering at J through a fog of medication, trying to fathom his slurred speech. He often seemed exhausted but could not be still. He would frequently ask to go to the toilet, or to refill his cup of water because of his dry mouth. Or he would stand up and start pacing in tiny circles in the confines of my small, narrow room. It was as though I was incarcerated with a prisoner pacing in a cramped cell. J seemed to perform a mad, disturbing dance. Mostly I found it impossible to think.

At one moment J would be in tears, at another moment telling me he felt he needed to cry, and at the same time he was trying to stop the tears. He would say he felt like screaming. He would accuse me of trying to seduce him. He would repeatedly insist the therapy was finished or that he should see a female therapist. He would talk about his plan of killing a policeman and, in frightening detail describe how he would get a gun to do it. Or he would talk of his determination to travel overseas, his resentment about the mental health tribunal and the police, who tried to stop him and take away his rights. He complained about the side effects of the medication, tingling sensations in his body and other disturbing reactions. Sometimes there was an involuntary twisting in his face, which I found unnerving. On some occasions he would be wearing necklaces, charms and talismans which he explained were to make him feel stronger. I found it hard to make sense of any of this, and hard to reach him. I felt as if I was in an antique, heavy diving suit trying to grasp a will-o'-the-wisp. Supervision was a sanctuary in which I was helped to see a weeping, screaming infant who felt in pieces, terrified of dissolving into tears, and was trying to stiffen himself in a desperate bid to hold himself together.

Just prior to the last of these four admissions there was an important development. J asked to see me before his scheduled appointment. He was aware he was breaking down and sought my help. Two weeks after the discharge from that admission, J came to a session asking if I would help him write a letter. These requests for help were surprising, he had not made any previous requests like this. He no longer seemed persecuted by me, and could turn to me for help. In subsequent sessions he took up a theme which continued through the following weeks and months: he kept trying to find a way of overcoming his difficulty in sleeping, because he was convinced his insomnia would lead to another breakdown. He discovered when he woke during the night it helped if he had something to eat, but he then worried about becoming overweight. J also complained of sleeping a lot during the day because of his poor sleep at night. He said he makes excuses for himself that he's making up for the years he didn't get much sleep, when he was working long shifts. He said he makes these excuses because he feels guilty about sleeping so much and being a lazy pig. At other times he spoke in a way that suggested some easing of the dominance of the psychotic superego. For example he talked about his need of the social security system in terms of what he described as the good and bad aspects of it. Over the next few weeks I started interpreting a baby in J who felt hungry and restless at night, who needed to be fed and comforted. J made no verbal response to these interpretations, but he would stretch out and make himself comfortable on his chair. We were sitting facing my desk and he found a way of bracing his feet against the side of the desk and of leaning back, eyes closed, with his head on the back of his chair, as though he were lying on a couch.

When we were approaching another break, as I gave J the dates there was a look of panic in his eyes. He came to the next session talking of someone who had sent him an e-mail with a virus which had wiped out some of his computer software, but it didn't wipe out the memory for his addresses and contacts. I said I thought when I gave him the news of the break it felt as though I was wiping him out, but he also wanted me to know he was able to hold onto a memory of a friendly contact with me. The more thoughtful atmosphere continued for the following weeks. I felt some hope about this next break. Just before the break he arrived for his session in a highly agitated state, again wearing various necklaces. I suggested he could see a colleague of mine during the holiday and he readily agreed. He told me he had made a detailed plan of activities for himself during the break when the rehab department would also be closed.

J managed to survive this break without being re-admitted, though I heard it was touch and go. When I saw him again he was calmer. I noticed he had put on some weight. He told me he was angry with the mental health tribunal for taking away his rights to travel. I said I thought he was angry with me too for going away, and not being able to stop me. He said he wasn't angry with me, after all he'd seen my colleague and it was good with her, why couldn't he continue seeing her? He yawned, stretched out and closed his eyes. He said he'd been sleeping a lot. He had woken during the previous night but was able to go back to sleep. He said he was aware of being high and of trying to keep himself down. He talked again about his fantasies of killing a policeman, which I linked with his anger about myself who left him. He insisted it was my prerogative to go away but agreed he felt it was unfair I could come and go as I please, whereas he did not have that freedom. He then asked why does he get high? I replied I thought a little fellow felt dropped when I go away, frightened of falling to pieces, and tries to hold himself together. As I said this he again stretched out, yawned and closed his eyes. The following week he came saying he had slept much better. He felt he was getting better, he did not have to take sleeping tablets to help him sleep. The next week this calm remained. He again found it helped him sleep when he had something to eat during the night. I talked about his hunger not just for food, but an emotional hunger. To my astonishment he replied: 'hungry for your food'. A little later he said he felt low. He was silent for a while. I asked him about his thoughts. He said he was wanting to leave because he had nothing more to say. I said I thought he was fearful I couldn't bear his sad feelings, or feelings he may not be able to put into words. He then spoke about his fears about the world coming to an end in a third world war. He said at first he thought it might be a little war, but with the biological virus weapons and so on, it's had an impact on him. This was a month after the twin towers attack of 9/11 in the US. It was the first reference J had made to those tragic events. It was an important development for him to be able to join in with others and share our fears. It was also a development for him to feel low and to tell me about it.

The next week he came with the familiar worries about sleeping and eating, worrying he would end up being twice his usual size. He reported a dream about a policeman watching him, watching his every move and waiting to see if he made a wrong move. J said he felt quite neutral in the dream and didn't feel frightened of the policeman. Later, after a silence he looked at me and, in an anguished voice, he told me how he sometimes thinks 'Oh no, I'm not going to recover, I'm not going to be as I used to be'. It was an intensely moving moment. I acknowledged how painful this thought was for him. In response he stretched out, yawned and seemed to sleep for a little while.

Whilst I could see J was indeed putting on weight, I thought he looked more solid, more substantial in a way that seemed to mirror his developing capacities to bear sad feelings. He remained troubled about his eating and I struggled to find a way of helping him to think about it. A few weeks later J spoke about a friend wanting him to take care of the new baby belonging to the friend's mistress. The friend urged J to make benefit claims for the baby, which J didn't want to do because it would be illegal. He said his friend is always up to some sort of monkey business. I acknowledged his disquiet about his friend. I went on to say because of our work together he was aware of a baby J who is hungry and restless and who needs my help. It's particularly difficult when he is on his own and having to care for this baby J by himself. He wonders what sort of monkey business I am up to showing him this baby to care for. He responded saying he was tired and exhausted. Near the end of this session, after a silence, he told me he hasn't visited the sex workers for several months, which was a record for him. I said I thought he was finding a different way of managing his feelings, but it was hard, tiring work. I felt we had finally found a way of talking about the baby J in a way that made sense to him, though he seemed somewhat suspicious about my motives in drawing his attention to the baby and what benefits I was seeking.

During the next session J found a new way of positioning himself in the chair. This time he rested his feet on the top corner of my desk, and lay back often closing his eyes as if he was lying in a hammock. He looked more at ease with his more substantial body. He told me since I last saw him he had slept deeply, and had a dream which felt very comfortable. He couldn't recall details of the dream but knew it was about the past. He looked so relaxed in this hammock position that, for a while, I thought he was falling asleep. He expressed concerns again about his eating at night, which he described as a craving. I said I thought it was a craving too for mental food, which he feels physically, a craving for food for thought to nourish his mind, to be understood so he could understand himself and his life; though this troubled him, it was after all an ordinary need for understanding. He agreed he did want to understand himself, and said 'So I shouldn't mind this craving for food?'. After a silence which seemed contemplative, he said on the internet talking to others is therapeutic, some of those he talks with are regulars. He gets to know them, talks about his life and his past. He said it's like taking some time off for a while so as to be able to move on. I agreed it sounded just like therapy. We were approaching the end of the session, rather wistfully he said it seems to have gone in a flash. Referring to the previous Christmas break, he said just a while ago it was coming up to 2000, and now it's 2001. As J could see, it was time for me to give him the next holiday dates and he was giving me my cue. We started preparing for another Christmas holiday.

Concluding Reflections on the Third Year

The improving contact with J toward the end of the second year, when he and I were able to think about a boy who needed to be understood, doubtless exacerbated the impact of that Christmas break. J began the third year in a precarious state. Nonetheless for a while we pursued some painful exploration of the damage he suffered because of psychosis. There was a poignant moment of contact when unusually J acknowledged a transference interpretation about my trying to control him. He sadly contemplated the implications of this understanding in seeing the damage he suffered from the influence of a psychotic superego in his withdrawal from others, who were condemned as trying to control him. Taking in this interpretation signalled a developing capacity to step back and observe himself. The projection about being controlled can be understood as a means of J trying to protect himself against fears of unintegration or fragmentation. The retrieval of the projection released him at that moment from a state of merger with me, and allowed a real contact with me as someone separate who could offer a different view. The awareness of separateness brought a real closeness which J sorely lacked. In the maternal transference he could feel held and understood. The unexpected cancellation of the following week's session because of my toothache, doubtless made him feel abruptly dropped. In the counter-transference I think the cancellation was an ache I experienced as a consequence of being in touch with his profound sadness, which I found hard to bear. The cancellation confirmed J's fear no-one could bear his longing to be held, or his sadness about loss.

J's subsequent breakdowns were precipitated by interruptions in the therapy. Following the breakdowns J again merged himself with me by a projective process in which my mind was taken over by beta elements, deadened and unable to think. I was frightened about his threats to kill a policeman. I could not think about the attacks on my mind in the transference to me as a policeman therapist; or see how his complaints that I was trying to seduce him reflected the invasiveness of his projections. Instead I was consumed by the experience of being in a cramped cell, controlled and held captive by the psychotic part of J's mind. While presenting sessions to my supervisor I was astonished and relieved she could think. When a link in my mind was re-established with a paternal psychoanalytic object it helped loosen the grip of J's projections on my mind as a maternal object, and I was able to start thinking again. As I regained more capacity to think during the sessions, unusually J asked for my help about the letter and so on. My supervisor said J was then apprehending me as a good object. He was able to apprehend me again as someone who could think about him, and help him feel understood in the maternal transference, a mother who could hold his infant self in mind. I was able to introduce a third figure, a newly appointed psychotherapist colleague who could be available for him during the holidays. J managed to survive the next break without an admission. He found a way of being held like an infant in a hammock, and he and I found a way of talking about the baby J. As my mind recovered in parallel, and perhaps because of my recovery, J recovered his mind.

For a while I became preoccupied with trying to understand the tormenting dance J kept performing in the confines of my office, as J spiralled into or out of psychosis. Returning to a paper by Britton (1992) titled 'Keeping things in mind', I was struck by a case example in which he described how the patient's father, because of his psychotic behaviour, had sabotaged the containment provided by the nursing couple of the patient's mother and his infant self. This insight gave me a way of thinking about J's mad dance. I thought perhaps he was showing me what it was like when he was being nursed by his mother and they were disturbed by his father, who suffered from psychosis. Similarly J and I were often disturbed by the psychotic part of J's mind. Later, when uncharacteristically, I tried making an historical interpretation in which I linked J's agitated state with disturbance in his early life, the interpretation seemed to mean nothing to J. More importantly, perhaps in arriving at this formulation I started thinking about J's projections, rather than being taken over by 'beta elements'.

When I was no longer identified with J's and my own fears about his anger, I could interpret his anger with me as helpful policeman therapist who left him when there was a break. J could later dream of a benign policeman who kept an eye on him. The dream confirms him apprehending me in the transference as a helpful observing paternal presence. I became an object with whom he could begin to identify. He sadly observed that the damage of his psychosis meant he could not be as he once was. When he could take in the policeman interpretation, his non-psychotic self owned some of his anger, a psychotic policeman father was less dominant in his mind, and there was a lessening of the psychotic superego's influence. An infant J was released into a maternal hammock cradle of the therapy; and an adult J could share in some of the depressive concerns of common humanity following 9/11.

References

Britton, R. (1989). The missing link: Parental sexuality in the Oedipus complex. In R. Britton et al. (Eds) *The Oedipus Complex Today*. London: Karnac.

Britton, R. (1992). Keeping things in mind. In R. Anderson (Ed.) *Clinical Lectures on Klein and Bion*. London: Routledge.

Caper, R. (1999). *A Mind of One's Own*. London: Routledge.

Chapter 8

Mourning Omnipotence – The Fourth Year of Therapy with J

Introduction

In the latter half of the fourth year a change in my personal life led to me giving notice to leave the unit, and needing to bring the therapy with J to an end. In the preceding six months there were most encouraging developments. J became involved in a meditation group in the local community. After the meditation sessions the group would have dinner together. This was the first time J mentioned any social interaction apart from activities organised by the rehabilitation unit. The woman, whom J described as his friend's 'mistress' and her baby, moved into the flat J shared with his mother. He began to make some good contact with her, and started referring to her by her first name, G. Sometimes he reported G making comments about his behaviour which shocked him, but he seemed to be taking in another perspective. He became more self-reflective, noticing things he tended to do when he got 'a bit high' or 'became ill'. He made tentative friendships with two other women. The consulting room began to feel full of people who were real and three dimensional. He was upset about putting on extra weight which was probably a side effect of his medication, though he also seemed to be hungrier and eating more. His new consultant psychiatrist agreed to reduce the medication. These developments brought a host of intense feelings, so much so I became worried J was on the verge of breaking down again. As I had several times previously, I offered him a second weekly session. Whereas before he refused such offers, this time he accepted. On the one hand attending more frequently intensified his feelings, especially a curiosity about myself and my life. On the other hand a second weekly session supported a more contemplative attitude towards himself and others, and he did not break down.

The Ending of the Therapy in the Fourth Year

It was with much regret that I anticipated ending the therapy with J. In the second week following a break during which I had made the decision to give notice, I told J I would be leaving the unit in three months' time. I said my

DOI: 10.4324/9781003319719-12

leaving did not coincide with his needs and, though he had done well, he would need to continue therapy. I said he could continue with my psychotherapist colleague whom he had seen when I was away. J's immediate response was to say he felt he had done a Bachelor's degree in Psychology with me, and he could now go on to a Masters with my colleague. In the next few weeks he brought much upset and disturbance. He became agitated and unable to sleep. He was preoccupied with anger about G because she was ignoring him. She resisted his attempts to get her to talk to him. He kept telling me about a photograph he had taken of her, and how he would cut it up, add different breasts and bum, and put it up for her to see. He returned to his preoccupation in the second year about trying to block incoming phone calls whose numbers were unidentified.

From a mixture of guilt and worry about J, for a while I tended to interpret too quickly and did not allow sufficient space for his despair. A dream and his associations from this period illustrates his experience of my difficulties. In the dream a woman was trying to clean up after a flood. When I asked him about the dream, he recalled G vacuuming the flat because the baby had dropped some food. He also spoke of reaching his megabyte limit in downloading from the internet. A friend had told him of a scheme whereby he could have unlimited downloading, but J felt sceptical about this. I said I thought he felt a flood of feelings about my leaving him but he felt there was a limit to what he could download on me, and perhaps he worried that was why I was leaving. Then, like the woman in the dream, he was left on his own to try to clean up feelings which he felt I could not bear, whereas he had expected an unlimited time with me. As he listened to this interpretation, he moved from a sitting position to one in which it was as if he was lying in a hammock. I took this hammock position as a confirmation the interpretation enabled him, especially his infant self, to feel held.

J continued to have problems sleeping. He came to his sessions red eyed, restless, almost in tears and worrying about cutting up G. He was also consumed with a photo of one of my occupational therapist colleagues he had taken. He had tried to photograph her as she was walking away from him. He called to her but, because she turned around too late, he photographed her back. He said when he showed her the photo it 'freaked her out'. He was contrite but also angry about it not being a way for a 'therapist' to behave. He said his mother told him he should stop coming to therapy because it was upsetting him too much. I said I was like a mother to him and with my leaving he felt all in pieces.

Before the next session somehow J discovered my hospital email address. He sent me an email message to pass on to the occupational therapist whom he had photographed. The message conveyed his anger about her reaction to the photograph. When he came to the session, he dismissed my interpretations linking his anger with me. He said if he was angry with me then he would be angry with all the doctors who had left over the years of his treatment in the hospital. This rebuttal confirmed how much hurt he felt not only about my leaving, but all the other leavings which he had suffered and felt unable to protest about. He also described a crescendo of feelings about cutting up G, so much so it appeared there were plans for G and her baby to move out of his flat. He was upset G might leave but also relieved because he was frightened about his murderous feelings about her.

J did not attend the next session. I was worried, tried phoning but he did not return my call. I prepared a message to send him. Later the same day I received a short email in which he wrote he wouldn't be seeing me anymore 'as i have lost confidence in u', the reasons for which he wrote 'i feel u know yourself'. He kept open the possibility of seeing my colleague after I had left. There was just a day before his next scheduled appointment so I decided to send an email reply. I wrote I understood his loss of confidence in me, in particular that he felt I could no longer cope with all his feelings about my leaving him. I wrote it wasn't helpful for him to stop at this time and I would keep his appointment times. J sent a reply before the next appointment, insisting he would not come back. He wrote he hoped he had not upset me in anyway. He did not attend the appointment. On the same day I sent a reply that it was because the therapy had been helping him that my leaving was so upsetting. I added in case he changed his mind I would keep his appointments for him. He replied the same day, writing 'nothing is going to change my mind'. He also asked if I had given the occupational therapist he'd photographed a copy of his email to her.

Willy nilly, unintentionally, I felt drawn into an email continuation of the therapeutic relationship for which I was ill prepared, never having done anything like it before. I was uneasy because I was not convinced by the literature which had started appearing about the value of email therapy. There were still six weeks before I was due to leave. Above all I felt it important to try to maintain contact with J and, if at all possible, to enable him to return for his remaining sessions. I was especially worried he might break down. I decided to wait until his next appointment in two days' time and send a reply during the session time. I deliberated whether or not to continue to interpret in this unfamiliar medium. I decided to take the risk. I wrote I thought he wanted me to know what it felt like when someone leaves suddenly and unexpectedly; he was angry with me as well as my colleague, but I felt he was worried about expressing his anger to me. I wrote he probably worried about spoiling a good contact, though not coming to his sessions was also a way of conveying his anger. J replied the same day, writing he was angry with me for reading the email he had sent for the occupational therapist, and not 'rejecting' it back to him. He wrote I was wasting my time by keeping the appointments for him. He asked me to give the time to 'someone in need'. I decided to continue this pattern of waiting until the next appointment and replying during the session. I also decided to continue to use the conventional writing style of sentences with complete spellings, punctuation and upper and lower case letters with which I felt comfortable, rather than the email vernacular of abbreviation and lower case which was popular and which J used.

I became worried J was becoming disturbed by my keeping appointments for him. My supervisor pointed out I needed to keep the appointments for myself to digest this ending. Five days later, during the next appointment, referring to his complaint about my reading the email to the occupational therapist, I wrote I thought J was angry with me for reading him in the way I had understood some of his feelings. He had allowed himself to get close to me and felt rejected by my leaving. I wrote I respected his position about not intending to return to his sessions, but I kept the appointments for both of us, for him and myself to work on the ending of an important relationship. J replied the same day. The subject of the email was 'good bye forever'. He wrote 'I will never never never come back'. He again added that he might continue with my colleague. He wrote he'd always wanted to finish with me but I kept 'pressuring him not to'. I felt alarmed by this reply because J seemed to feel persecuted by me. I wasn't sure how to respond without increasing the persecution. I felt completely at sea in this medium of emails and was just kept afloat by my supervisor. I decided not to reply during the next appointment but to wait and think, just as one might in a session.

I didn't know what to do. I was worried J could expect me to retaliate by giving up on him, and certainly I did feel exasperated. I thought it important to let him know at least I was still holding him in mind. A week later, during the next appointment I replied simply thanking him for his message and that I was 'thinking about' his message. In discussions with my supervisor I came to appreciate, albeit reluctantly, that I needed to accept in all likelihood J would not return to the consulting room; and that my leaving might well precipitate another breakdown. At least he had managed to come this far and stay in contact with me via email. I began to hear some worrying accounts from my occupational therapy colleagues that J was sometimes talking in a bizarre way. There was an angry exchange at the gym between J and one of the male occupational therapists. Later, an anonymous letter was sent to this colleague complaining about his behaviour, it was suspected J was its author. J wrote to the head of the rehabilitation department saying he thought it was time for him to 'graduate from the rehab'. He also apologised for writing to the female occupational therapist to complain about her reaction to the photograph.

Another psychiatrist took over J's case earlier than anticipated because of staff changes in the hospital. The new consultant, whom I had not met, arranged to see J with a view to possible admission. The consultant concluded J did not need to be admitted. The occupational therapists were worried about J but, unlike previous times when he had talked in ways they found frightening, this time he expressed his anger and grievances in a way they could see was connected with the impact of my leaving. I saw my task as to try to keep in touch with him, and help him continue to express his feelings rather than lose his mind.

I waited and did not send or receive any message from J during the next two appointments. In the third appointment, which was nine days since my previous 'thinking about your message' email, I wrote simply: 'I am wondering how you are? I would be pleased to hear from you'. J replied the next day. He wrote he was 'not too bad'. He described being upset with the female occupational therapist he had photographed. He finished with the statement he should now stand on his own two feet. I felt relieved by the reply because his sense of persecution seemed diminished. I was particularly encouraged by the moderateness of the 'not too bad' description of himself.

I was troubled there was something I was failing to understand in J's recurring reference to the photograph of my colleague, and discussed it again with my supervisor. My supervisor talked of the importance of the mother's face, an infant wanting a glimpse of mother's face and J's feeling he had chased me away because he wanted so much more from me. In my reply during the next appointment I wrote perhaps I had not understood his appreciative feelings, and that he might feel I was leaving because I could not bear his longing to feel close and understood. I concluded 'I wonder what you think about these thoughts?' J replied the same day, writing he didn't 'quite understand'. He then described worries connected with trying to start some work again as a hairdresser. It seemed he had placed an advertisement in a local paper but worried he wouldn't have the energy if a job came up. At the following appointment, wanting to encourage him I wrote this was a hard and testing time, and I thought he was managing well.

There were just two weeks left before my departure. J's emails became longer, more detailed and more like the way he talked in the sessions. He was especially pleased because he had acquired some software which enabled him to screen out unidentified phone calls, and his psychiatrist had reduced his lithium medication. He sent me a copy of an angry letter he had written to G. I replied simply that I could understand him feeling angry and it was good he was expressing his feelings. In the penultimate week I wrote to remind him I would be leaving at the end of the next week. His reply on the same day conveyed a sense of shock. He asked if this was the end of the 'email therapy' and whether he would need to see my colleague. Concerned by J's sense of panic, I decided to reply on the same day even though I would be replying outside the appointment time. I wrote I felt he needed to continue the therapy with my therapist colleague. Almost by return J replied indicating he would see my colleague, and he would judge for himself whether to continue with her.

In the penultimate session I wrote I was glad he would see my colleague. I thanked him for working with me. I wrote I thought we had done some very good work together, it had been a privilege to work with him. I added I would be pleased to know how things went for him. If he wanted to write to me, letters sent to the hospital would be forwarded to me. J replied on the same day telling me he felt 'empowered' because of his software which screened out the unidentified callers. He described 'good news' that he had done his 'very first paid hairdressing job', and added 'though it was for a good friend and i charged her less'. During the last session I sent my congratulations, acknowledging he had made considerable achievements in other ways too. I concluded 'I shall miss seeing you'. J sent a final reply with its email subject 'miss u too'. He wrote he was attaching a photograph, 'the best pic i have taken'. Indeed it was a charming photograph of him. I was deeply touched.

Concluding Reflections

Ending the therapy with J brought a fear for him and myself that he would collapse into a psychotic state. The fear reflected our experience of his breakdowns which were often precipitated by interruptions in the therapy. He had not suffered a breakdown since he started attending twice weekly and the arrangement for my psychotherapist colleague to see him during the breaks. The timing of the ending was unfortunate, to say the least, because it was only a short while since he began attending twice weekly, and giving just three months' notice was minimal. He was terribly hurt and felt sorely rejected. His anger and hurt were displaced onto G and two of my occupational therapy colleagues in the rehabilitation service. He needed to preserve a good relationship with me and could only manage by splitting in this way. The precariousness of this defence was evident when my emails became persecuting to him.

A turning point occurred when I accepted J probably would not return to the consulting room and might well break down. Neville Symington (1983) has written about how an 'inner act of freedom' in the therapist can promote 'a therapeutic shift in the patient'. I understand this shift comes about because the therapist relinquishes using projective identification to possess and control the patient. Caper has described how therapists can be drawn to trying to influence the patient's mind by projective identification. Following Freud, Caper understands there is often a transference which involves a desire for a healer, with a consequent pressure in the counter-transference which may meet a corresponding wish to heal. Caper points out therapists are vulnerable to this kind of healer transference because it can hook into our wish to deny our sadism and destructiveness (1999). Winnicott has written of hate in the counter-transference (1949) which can be expressed in the ending of the session; and hate can be conveyed in the ending of a therapy, especially in such a relatively abrupt ending as mine with J. Caper sees that the awareness of our destructive impulses gives an additional meaning to psychoanalytic containment: to contain a patient analytically therapists must first contain their anxieties about their destructive impulses which are defended against by beliefs about the omnipotence of psychoanalysis (1999, p. 31).

I did not complete the paper on which this chapter is based until seven years after the therapy ended. Undoubtedly my considerable guilt about ending the therapy contributed to problems in mourning and the long time it took for me in the writing. The task for J and myself was to mourn the ending, which James Fisher (2000) described as a 'mourning in the presence of a loved object'. Fisher was referring to the 'agony that resides in the psychic reality that the object is outside of my control and my ability to possess it', which he quoted Donald Meltzer described as the 'enigmatic' quality of the loved one. Drawing on the work of Bion and Meltzer, Fisher elucidates this process in Shakespeare's tragedy of King Lear in Lear's attempts to be a good father to his daughters, seeking to bribe them to love him by abdicating and endowing them their inheritance. Fisher writes:

'It is as if Lear senses but can never quite realize a knowing, a desire to understand, that can acknowledge the freedom of the loved object. As a father he could not trust that he might be loved, and of course might also not be loved – this is the anxiety that comes with the reality that love is a gift, a gift that may or may not be given. His perversion of 'endowing' into an abdication, which appeared to make the daughters' inheritance a gift, disguised the reality that what he sought was possession and control of children. It was in that sense the opposite of endowing' (2000, p. 980).

Fisher sees acknowledging the freedom of the object means mourning our omnipotence 'since its freedom is not within our gift'. It also means mourning 'an intimacy which was an illusion' because of the need to possess and control, and which avoided a painful 'uncertainty, the not-knowing whether or when the freedom to go separate ways will also be a freedom to come together again. Intimacy is the gift of that freedom' (2000, p. 977).

Peter Hildebrand (2001) wrote a courageous account about how, when he discovered he was dying from a terminal illness, he had to prematurely conclude his analysis of a much disturbed young woman. Hildebrand drew inspiration from his study of Shakespeare's *The Tempest*. He felt identified with Prospero's 'painful acceptance of his own anger and pain at the loss of the island and his capacity to contemplate the imminence of his own death' (2001, p. 1244). Hildebrand observes that the paucity of literature about 'the impact of the disappearance or death of the analyst on his/her patients' shows how difficult it is for the analyst, like Prospero, 'to give up his powers'. Hildebrand also drew on Lacan's idea that the patient treats the analyst as 'the person who will know and be able to cure what is wrong with him or her'. Hildebrand points out this is an 'assumption which all patients have to painfully surrender in order to effect a cure and take control over their own lives and their inner worlds as much as is possible' (2001, p. 1244). These insights echo Caper's ideas about the patient's transference on to the therapist as an omnipotent healer, and are a reminder that in mourning separation in therapy, both patient and therapist need to be able to retrieve projective identifications from each other.

When I was trying to influence J to return to the consulting room for his remaining sessions I was enacting an omnipotent phantasy in projective identification that I could invade his mind and control it. This doubtless contributed to J's escalating persecutory state. My supervisor helped me step back, recognise my helplessness and J's separateness. When I sent the email saying I was thinking it over, with the help of a third perspective there was now a triangular space in which to think (Britton, 1989), and interestingly J's persecutory state diminished. Even more remarkable, for a patient who often retreated into mania rather than feel sad, when we reached the end of what J described as 'the email therapy' he was able to bear some pain of loss, acknowledged in the 'miss u too' email. He attached a good photo of himself which suggests he felt in touch with loved and loving internal objects. Perhaps the move to an exchange of emails was a first step for both of us in separating, but staying in touch. Perhaps this online technology contributed to J facing the ending and bearing some depressive feelings without breaking down.

Being able to mourn brings painful feelings of sadness, sorrow and guilt because it means recognising separateness, destructiveness and helplessness. If these feelings can be borne, then the lost loved ones can be established internally in a symbolical way which also recognises their loss, and in a way which enriches our internal world. We need to be able to mourn our omnipotence in relation to the objects in our internal world, which Caper (1987) describes as accepting these internal objects have lives of their own, and passionate relationships with one another that one can only observe without being part of, or controlling. For Caper this means an acceptance that one's mind has a life of its own, and passions one can only observe and know about without controlling (1997, p. 54).

A post script

I sometimes wondered whether there would be some objection from staff in the unit about my seeing J for long term once and latterly twice weekly therapy. I had been given an open brief but therapeutic resources were scarce. By contrast when I began my career in psychology, over forty years earlier, there were many residential and day hospital therapy services, as well as plentiful outpatient therapy, all provided by the public health service. In the changed, much reduced context in which I was conducting the therapy with J, there were no objections about the length or frequency of my therapy with him from my colleagues, including the nursing staff on the ward where J was re-admitted on the occasions he broke down during the therapy. I think my colleagues were relieved to see J receiving the therapy he so much needed, and from which he was slowly benefitting. Some months after my therapy ended with J, I heard that he continued to see my psychotherapist colleague. For a while the therapy went well but my colleague became very ill and had to resign from her post. Her post was not immediately replaced. I later heard the rehabilitation staff were again worried about J.

J is an example of someone I believe needs long term, perhaps even lifelong therapeutic help. I hope I have demonstrated how therapy helped him begin to achieve a more fulfilling life. The continuing reduction and undermining of therapeutic and other welfare services for patients like J, reflects societies which have become dominated by what Rosenfeld (1971) described as destructive narcissism. David Bell, in a paper titled 'Primitive mind of state', drawing on Rosenfeld's work, presciently described how attacks on welfare provision gain support from appealing to primitive parts of the personality, a destructive narcissism which hates vulnerability and dependency (Bell, 1996). The antagonism against providing help for vulnerable people is often fuelled by propaganda of pejorative descriptions of such people as scroungers, skivers or shirkers. I retain some hope from my experience of teaching about therapy to some of the increasing numbers of people who, despite the negative propaganda and assaults on therapy provision, proceed to pursue trainings in what Freud called an 'impossible profession'.

References

Bell, D. (1996). Primitive mind of state. *Psychoanalytic Psychotherapy, 10* (1), 45–57.

Britton, R. (1989). The missing link: Parental sexuality in the Oedipus complex. In R. Britton et al. (Eds) *The Oedipus Complex Today*. London: Karnac.

Caper, R. (1997). Symbol formation and creativity. In D. Bell (Ed.) *Reason and Passion*. London: Routledge.

Caper, R. (1999). *A Mind of One's Own*. London: Routledge.

Fisher, J. (2000). A father's abdication: Lear's retreat from aesthetic conflict. *International Journal of Psychoanalysis, 81*, 963–82.

Hildebrand, P. (2001). Prospero's paper. *International Journal of Psychoanalysis, 82*, 1235–46.

Rosenfeld, H. (1971). A clinical approach to the psychoanalytic theory of the life and death instincts: An investigation into the aggressive aspects of narcissism. *International Journal of Psychoanalysis, 52*, 169–78.

Symington, N. (1983). The analyst's act of freedom as agent of therapeutic change. *International Review of Psychoanalysis, 10*, 283–91.

Winnicott, D.W. (1949). Hate in the counter-transference. *International Journal of Psychoanalysis, 30*, 69–74.

Part IV

Life

The following shorter chapters offer illustrations of how psychoanalytic concepts, which informed my approach to the clinical work in the previous chapters, helped me in thinking about social and political life.

DOI: 10.4324/9781003319719-13

Chapter 9

War

This chapter offers some reflections about war which were stimulated by the film *No Man's Land* released in 2001 about the Bosnian war. The screenplay was written by the film's director Danis Tanovic.

A Precis of *No Man's Land*

The film opens with a scene of soldiers lost in a fog. They are a relief group of Bosnian soldiers making their way to the front line. They make jokes about their guide's incompetence. He advises them to wait until dawn when the fog will clear. At dawn the fog lifts to reveal a beautiful rural landscape. The Bosnians discover they are in front of the Serbian lines. There is a sudden barrage of gunfire, after which it seems they are all killed. Two Serbian soldiers are sent to investigate. They search the trench in between the two lines – the no man's land. One of them drags an apparently dead Bosnian soldier on top of a mine which he sets so it will explode if the body is moved. Tchicki, a Bosnian who has survived, kills one of these two Serbian soldiers and wounds the other, Nino. Tchicki orders Nino to strip and walk along the outside of the trench waving a white cloth. Both sides are thrown into confusion by this sight because they cannot identify which side Nino is from. The trench is blasted with gunfire. As Nino and Tchicki shelter from the gunfire they break into a fierce argument about whose side started the war. At gunpoint Tchicki forces Nino to say his side started it.

They discover that Tchicki's friend and comrade, Tsera, who was laid on top of the mine, is in fact alive. As Tchicki bends over to help him Nino grabs a gun and takes control. Nino points the gun at Tchicki and asks who started the war? Tchicki is forced to say his side did. Later, when Tsera asks for a cigarette and Nino goes to give him one, Tsera traps him. The impasse is only resolved when they agree to both have guns. 'We are equal now', Nino says. For a while there is a conversation between them in which they become amused to discover that a former girlfriend of Tchicki was a classmate of Nino.

DOI: 10.4324/9781003319719-14

Nino then suggests they both strip and walk along the outside of the trenches waving white cloths. Both sides are thrown into further consternation, they cannot identify these men and are not even sure whether the men are soldiers or civilians. Both sides call up a United Nations group in the locality. It is led by a Frenchman Marchand, who is fed up with helplessly watching and decides to go in without awaiting further orders. When he reports what he finds there to his superiors he is immediately ordered out. He offers to take Nino and Tchicki with him. Tchicki refuses to leave Tsera and shoots Nino to wound him so he cannot leave. Nino inflamed with hatred vows to kill Tchicki.

As the UN team leaves, they are intercepted by a television news crew which is led by a woman reporter. She has listened to the conversation Marchand had with his superiors. Marchand talks to her about the role of the UN. He says he feels standing by doing nothing is taking sides. He lets her speak to his superiors. With Marchand's encouragement she insists the UN send the team back, and agree to send in a bomb disposal expert. When the UN team arrives at the trench again, they are just in time to prise Nino from Tchicki, whom he is about to stab with Tchicki's knife. Tchicki is furious and vows to kill Nino.

Meanwhile, the head of the UN mission is apoplectic with rage because against his orders the UN has been drawn in. Accompanied by a blonde miniskirted assistant he lands at the trench by helicopter. The bomb disposal expert concludes nothing can be done to dismantle the mine. There is a shoot-out between Tchicki and Nino who had been ordered to leave the trench. Tchicki kills Nino and Tchicki is killed by a UN soldier. All of this is filmed by the television crew as a stunned studio director looks at the screens. Earlier this same director had urged his team to interview the soldiers, including the soldier lying on top of the mine. The head of the UN tells the media the mine has been defused, the soldier who was laid on top of it is in a critical condition and being taken out by the helicopter. As they all depart the scene, the film ends with a final view of the trench where Tsera lies alone on top of the mine.

Some Reflections

Early in the film when Tchicki and Nino shelter from the gunfire caused by Nino's appearance outside the trench, they briefly lament the destruction of the beautiful landscape. Then an argument breaks out about whose side started the war and violated the land. It is almost comic how Tchicki wins the argument by insisting at gunpoint that Nino admit it was Nino's side started the war; and then later, when Nino has overpowered Tchicki and has the gun, he forces Tchicki to admit it was Tchicki's side. A brief moment of sorrow is followed by an insistence of the other side's destructiveness and guilt, ironically by murderous threats indicative of mutual projections of destructiveness between the two men and the two sides.

As the story develops, we see how this projective process between the warring sides is enacted between the two men as they develop a murderous hatred for each other, which finally results in their deaths. Nino hates Tchicki for stopping him leaving with the UN, taking away his freedom to escape. Nino's phantasy of being able to evacuate his own destructiveness into Tchicki is what diminishes his freedom because the projection possesses and controls his mind. Tchicki's hatred of Nino for trying to kill him with Tchicki's own knife, contains a projection of Tchicki's own murderous feelings which the knife represents, and which ultimately are the source of his own death. The two men become locked together not only in physical combat, but also in a mutual projective process, and the projections hook into destructive aspects in each other's personality. This projective process is accompanied by superegos, which take the moral high ground and fuel a condemnation of destructiveness attributed to the other.

The two men and the two sides are merged together in a projective process, in essence suffering from mutual evacuations. Their own murderousness is felt to be in the other side which is condemned for it. It suggests harsh, ruthless superegos. Such internal objects are more likely to arise as a result of severe trauma, especially when the infant or child has been exposed to terrifying experiences; and when the means of managing those experiences is to create within the mind an equally terrifying figure or gang, to hold the self together in the face of such assaults. The more frightening the trauma, the more frightening the internal structure created to manage it. Some of the worst and most prolonged wars can be seen to breed on long histories of relentless horror and devastation.

When I was thinking about the film, I heard a performance of some of Monteverdi's madrigals of love and war composed in 1638. The strange coupling of love and war inspired this beautiful and sensuous music. One of the madrigals is about two warrior knights fighting until one finally kills the other, only to tragically discover the dead warrior is his lover whose identity was obscured by armour. Two lovers locked in each other's embrace are not so different from two warriors locked in combat. Lovers also suffer from delusions, though benign and delightful ones in which they projectively merge, attributing loved and loving qualities to each other. The loved one for a while becomes an idealized extension of oneself, just as the hated warrior comes to represent all that is hated and hating in oneself, and may thus become an external embodiment of internal persecutors.

Mediation is attempted in the film by the intervention of a UN soldier who understands that doing nothing is not necessarily neutral, because it may be a way of taking sides. He tries to do something and is assisted by the media. I think this quest for peace in the film recognises the need for a third party, a third view which is not taken over by the mutual projective delusions, and which can help the two sides separate and see themselves for who they are. Indeed, the first softening of the relationship between Nino and Tchicki comes about through their discovered relationship with a former girlfriend and classmate, which in a moment of humour gives them a friendly view of each other. However, as the UN soldier comes to appreciate, when the third party has vested interests the third party is no longer neutral. The UN and the media are shown to have such interests which obstruct a helpful intervention. Third parties are especially vulnerable to taking sides when they wish to deny their own sadism. When third parties want to insist only on their virtuousness they will be inclined to join in attributing destructiveness to one or both sides, and the measures taken to achieve peace may well enact denied hatred belonging to the third party. For example, I think that vested interests in peace brokers, who want to deny their own destructiveness and export it elsewhere, contribute to the failure of peace interventions in the Middle East. Often the effects of the sanctions used in efforts to achieve peace, betray an underlying murderousness in those who devise and apply the sanctions.

Peace, I believe, can come only from an acknowledgement of one's own destructiveness and an attempt to manage it as best one can, often not knowing what the outcome will be. Hence, I see the final image in the film as a poignant reminder that in the end we, like Tsera, are alone with the explosive potential of our own destructiveness, a potential to destroy ourselves and those whom we love.

Chapter 10

The Holocaust

Stefan Zweig's novel *Beware of Pity* led me to thinking about envy and the Holocaust. Zweig completed the novel in 1938 and published it in 1939. He was a highly successful Jewish writer who left Austria in 1934 and went to London where he wrote this book, his only full length novel. Apprehensive about internment he left London in 1939, travelled to the USA and then Brazil where he remained. The novel begins on the cusp of the Second World War when the narrator reports a story told to him by an Austrian cavalry officer about his life during the period leading up to the First World War. In the 2011 English translation of the novel, there is a foreword by Nicholas Lezard who describes how in exile Zweig was reluctant to make any statements about the treatment of the Jews in Nazi Germany. Lezard suggests, though the novel could seem somewhat nostalgic for pre-First World War Austria, Zweig chose to comment obliquely. Lezard sees the novel as a warning to 'not judge things by appearances'. I shall pursue this theme to discuss how Zweig's novel unmasks what appears to be pity to reveal an envious superego in the Austrian cavalry officer, which destroys a Jewish man and his daughter. Moreover, I see the novel as a conscious or unconscious warning from Zweig about how such envy, mobilised in the social conditions of privation and fear prior to the Second World War, contributed to the Holocaust.

A Precis of the Novel

The cavalry officer Anton's story begins when he was aged twenty-five, stationed in a small garrison town on the Hungarian border. He becomes acquainted with the rich widowed Hungarian Herr von Kekesfalva and his disabled daughter Edith. Anton presumes they are aristocrats. Edith is unable to walk as a result of a riding accident. Anton is consumed with pity. He becomes a regular visitor to their home, a magnificent villa where he savours their lavish hospitality. He learns that Kekesfalva is a Jew from an impoverished beginning, who made a fortune and bought his aristocratic title. Out of pity Anton gives Kekesfalva and Edith false hope that their physician

DOI: 10.4324/9781003319719-15

Dr Condor believes a new treatment could cure the paralysis of her legs. In fact Dr Condor is not at all convinced that the treatment will be successful. Anton becomes aware Edith has fallen in love with him. He is shocked. He takes flight to Dr Condor, who helps him find the resolve to support Edith's attempt at the treatment. Anton returns to the Kekesfalva villa, realises his affection for Edith and agrees to marry her at the completion of the treatment. There is a celebratory dinner, after which he encounters some of his cavalry comrades who confront him with a rumour of his betrothal. He denies the engagement. Later he is consumed with self-disgust and plans suicide. He is persuaded by his commandant to be transferred to another garrison. En route he has second thoughts, sends Edith an apologetic telegram reassuring her about his love, and leaves a message seeking Dr Condor's help. The assassination of Archduke Franz Ferdinand at Sarajevo, which precipitated the First World War, obstructs the telegram being delivered to Edith, and prevents Dr Condor from reaching her before she commits suicide. Her father dies a few days later. Anton is devastated, ridden with guilt, takes flight into the war and becomes a much decorated hero. At the conclusion of the novel, attending a performance of an opera Anton finds himself sitting next to Dr Condor. Full of shame, he scuttles away in the dark before Condor can recognise him.

Some Reflections

Early in the novel, Anton notices what he describes as his 'first symptom of poisoning by pity' during an exhilarating morning gallop with his squadron. He imagines the crippled Edith watching and envying his physical prowess. He feels overcome with pity for her, reins in his horse and orders his men to a slow trot. It is only when he is out of sight of the Kekesfalva villa that he remonstrates with himself to 'stop wallowing in sentimentality', and orders his men to resume the gallop. I understand Anton to be trying to rein in his envy by denying it in his pity and projectively attributing it to Edith. However, he recognises his pity is sentimental and poisonous, which reminds me of how Winnicott (1949) described sentimentality as a denial of hatred. In this sentimental pity the envy seeps through.

Zweig knew Freud well and continued to visit him when they were both in exile in London. In the novel, Anton and Dr Condor show impressive capacities for self reflection which suggest the influence of Zweig's relationship with Freud. Anton, in conflict about his sentimental pity, describes an internal dialogue between two voices, one urges him to return to the Kekesfalva villa and the other warns him against it. When he receives an invitation for dinner from Kekesfalva, which indicates there will be certain military dignitaries present, he readily accepts. At the dinner he imagines his comrades in the garrison envying his presence at the gathering. I understand the internal dialogue as a conflict between an envious superego that is drawn to the contacts and riches Kekesfalva can provide, and an ego that rightly apprehends that sentimental pity will get him into trouble. But his envy is denied, project-ively attributed to his comrades, and introjected into his superego, which is thereby strengthened and able to dominate the ego's better judgement.

When Anton admits to Dr Condor that, from pity, he gave Kekesfalva and Edith false hope the new treatment would cure her, Dr Condor warns Anton that pity can become a 'murderous poison'. Condor describes two kinds of pity, the sentimental sort which tries to rid oneself of the pain of the sufferer, and the unsentimental kind which 'knows its own mind and is determined to stand by the sufferer, patiently suffering too'. I think the pain, which a sentimental pity tries to evacuate, is a pain about envy which is projectively attributed to the sufferer, whose vulnerability for envying the wellbeing of others may provide a ready hook for such projections. The unsentimental kind of pity Condor describes indicates an ego with the strength to bear taking responsibility for its envy, and out of concern to identify empathically with the pain of the sufferer.

When Anton discovers that Edith loves him, he is overcome with revul-sion that this 'imperfectly formed, helpless creature' had the audacity to love like a 'real woman'. Dr Condor warns him that to abandon Edith, after she has opened her heart to him and is about to try the new treatment, would be to murder her. In a Freudian guise, Condor then interprets Anton's response to her love as his fear of being mocked and looking ridiculous in front of others, especially his military comrades. Anton confirms the accuracy of this interpretation:

> 'I felt that Condor had driven a sharp, thin needle into my heart. For what he described was what I had felt, unconsciously, for a long time, only I had not dared to think of it ... as soon as I was aware of Edith's passionate love my principal feeling had been of shame in front of others'.
>
> (Zweig 2011, p. 344)

Condor supports Anton in standing up to the fear of mockery and shame. Anton's experience finds echoes in Condor's own, having married a blind woman and withstanding the disapprobation of his mother and his colleagues. Anton witnesses the loving relationship between Dr Condor and his wife which further strengthens him in his determination to return to Edith and support her in the new treatment.

Condor's interpretation gives Anton a view of a mocking, envious superego which is projectively attributed to others. When Anton is thereby enabled to observe his mind, for a while he is not so dominated by the superego. Witnessing the loving relationship between Dr Condor and his wife, prob-ably supports a loving internal couple and Anton's loving feelings. Anton returns to Edith but his resolve wavers. Again out of pity, he makes a pledge to Kekesfalva to marry Edith if the outcome of the treatment is successful. To his surprise he finds Edith quite changed as a result of this pledge. Instead of a crippled girl whom he feels is trying to manipulate him, he feels in the presence of a woman who truly loves him, insisting she will only marry him if she is cured because she does not want to burden him with her disability. Anton then feels in touch with a tenderness for Edith and willingly confirms the betrothal. He is soon assailed with misgivings. He is especially fearful of his Aunt Daisy's reaction to him for bringing Jews into the family and dishonour upon his regiment. He has a dream of his family ridiculing him for becoming engaged to a rich heiress who is disabled. The dream reveals a cruel internal gang, the envious superego.

A pivotal episode in the novel is when Anton meets some of his comrades who challenge him about the rumour of his engagement. He fears if he were to admit the engagement, they would mock him. When he denies the engagement, his comrades praise him for not bringing dishonour and shame upon the regiment. He remains silent while they continue to pour abuse on Kekesfalva and Edith. To himself he admits:

> 'I am horribly aware that with my silence I have wickedly, murderously let that poor, innocent girl down ... I had let my comrades abuse her father without a word of protest'.
>
> (pp. 413–14)

In his fear of his comrades' reaction to the engagement Anton projectively attributes the envious superego, mocking gang to his comrades, who have ready hooks for such projections in their hatred of Jews. Anton's ego is as incapable of standing up to the comrades in the external world, as it is to the superego gang in his internal world. His ego is depleted as a result of the denial of hatred in his sentimentality, and by the projection of his envy which, when introjected, strengthens his envious superego. His later decision to commit suicide shows the destructiveness of his superego turning against his ego. His commanding officer's intervention supports his ego to fight against the superego's suicidal exhortations, and enables him to be in touch with his ego's concern for Edith. He writes a letter for Condor to give Edith, in which for the first time he is able to acknowledge and give expression to his love for her. Melanie Klein saw how love can mitigate envy. For Anton, it is too late. The outbreak of the war and its destructiveness prevents Anton's attempts to save Edith, and leads to an enactment of his murderous envy towards Edith and her father.

In the ending of the novel, the opera at which Anton finds himself sitting next to Dr Condor is Gluck's 'Orpheus'. Anton is drawn to the 'pure, restrained melancholy' in this opera about Orpheus who suffered the bereavement of his beloved Eurydice, and tries to retrieve her from Hades. This story alludes to Anton's melancholia and a persecuting guilt from which he feels no escape, conveyed in the novel's closing sentence '... no guilt is forgotten while the conscience still remembers it'. This is the destructive superego masquerading as a conscience. Stefan Zweig probably had first-hand acquaintance with such a superego. In 1942, just four years after the completion of the novel, Zweig and his wife Lotte committed suicide. Lotte was his second wife whom he said he married out of pity.

I see this novel as a prescient warning from Zweig about the dreadful persecution and murder of Jews during the Second World War. The novel reveals envy of the Jews as an important motive in the persecutors and murderers in the Holocaust, and how denial of envy and hatred probably contributed to the silence and inaction of many others who were aware of the persecution and slaughter.

References

Winnicott, D.W. (1949). Hate in the counter-transference. *International Journal of Psychoanalysis, 30,* 69–74.

Zweig, S. (2011). *Beware of Pity* (A. Bell, Trans.). London: Pushkin.

Chapter 11

Entitlement

On first reading Alan Bennett's *The Uncommon Reader* (2006) about Queen Elizabeth II's transformation when she becomes an avid reader, I enjoyed it as a whimsical piece of satire. Returning to it I came to appreciate Bennett's beautifully crafted work has much more to offer. I saw Bennett offering a commentary about a society characterised by entitlement and corruption.

A Precis of the Novel

The novel begins with the Queen at a state banquet asking a reluctant French President about Jean Genet. The President is not amused. He thinks to himself he is in a 'for a long evening'. The novel's narrator then traces the history of the Queen's enthusiasm for literature, beginning when she comes across a travelling library parked behind the kitchens at Buckingham Palace. Curious, she ventures in and meets the driver librarian and the one reader Norman, who works in the royal kitchens. Out of politeness she feels obliged to borrow a book. She ends up picking a book by Ivy Compton-Burnett, whom she remembers making a Dame. Thus begins a new-found love affair with reading, initially with Norman as her guide and mentor. Norman, who is gay, is subsequently promoted as a page to the Queen. The Queen reads widely and prodigiously. Her Majesty's reading is not well received. Her courtiers complain she is neglecting her appearance. Worse still, when she goes on walkabouts and meets her people, she stops asking the routine questions such as how they travelled there that day, for which they have been prepared and can give routine answers. Instead she asks her subjects what they are reading, and sometimes even hands out books she herself has finished.

The Prime Minister becomes especially fed up when, during his regular audiences with the Queen, she starts drawing on her growing study of history in order to quiz him about his own acquaintance with the history of some of the countries in which his government is intervening. She finds him lacking in such knowledge and suggests texts he read, which he strongly resents. Various attempts are made to discourage the Queen's reading. For example,

DOI: 10.4324/9781003319719-16

books she selected to accompany an overseas visit go missing. During one of her absences overseas, Norman is removed. An old, now retired royal retainer is sent to talk her out of reading. Such efforts to sabotage her reading fail. Nonetheless the Queen tends to become discouraged by feeling she has no voice of her own. She also starts to become aware of other people's feelings in a way she had not previously considered. She notices a courtier has become embarrassed and confused by something she has said; she realises, when she comes across Norman again, that he is resentful and hurt by the way he was removed. She becomes preoccupied with what she has missed in life and feels sad about it.

The coup de théâtre occurs in the final chapter. The Queen summons all her mentors and advisors, including former prime ministers and members of the government to a gathering during the year of her 80th birthday. She announces she has decided to try her hand at writing about her life, which she feels needs 'redeeming by analysis and reflection'. To the increasing discomfort, particularly of the government, she starts musing aloud about how, during the course of her reign, she has met and entertained visiting heads of state some of them 'unspeakable crooks and blackguards'; and how at times she has 'been forced to participate if only passively in decisions I consider ill-advised and often shameful'. She has felt monarchy is 'just a government-issue deodorant'. Her audience is by now alarmed. The Prime Minister triumphantly reminds the Queen that her unique position as monarch would prevent her from publishing such a book. The Queen responds citing examples of her predecessors who have done so, lastly including her uncle the Duke of Windsor and his book *A King's Story*. The Prime Minister points out that the book could only have been written because the Duke had abdicated. The Queen plays her trump card saying 'Oh, did I not say that? ... Why do you think you're all here?'

Some Reflections

In his paper on narcissism, Freud (1914) first used the phrase 'His Majesty the Baby' to evoke an omnipotent state of mind that characterises narcissism in infancy. Tuckett and Taffler (2008) return to this phrase in discussing the volatility of the stock market in financial crises of the West. They use 'His Majesty the Baby' to illustrate narcissism of paranoid-schizoid states of mind which can recur throughout life. The authors see such narcissism is fuelled by omnipotent phantasies of limitless financial rewards, excitement and greed. In such states of mind, the financiers and their customers who were caught up in financial bubbles of such enterprises as the dot.com companies, were able to ignore unpalatable facts about the precariousness of those enterprises. Later, when the same enterprises crashed, guilt was denied and projectively attributed to convenient scapegoats.

Bernardine Bishop (2001) in a psychoanalytic study of Lear and Prospero in Shakespeare's plays, points out that in our struggles to achieve maturity such royal figures can be a metaphor 'for whatever sense we may have of our share of responsibility for the world; for acceptance of the unchosen in our lives – that what we are born into also belongs to whom we are' (p. 506). She sees the attainment of these goals may 'only be apparent' and not real, because of the absence of internal growth due to an incapacity to face depressive pain. Consequently, royal status may confirm 'entitlement to infantile aims' and encourage 'ownership and omnipotence'. Bishop shows how Lear remains stuck in an infantile state, whereas Prospero develops and is able to relinquish omnipotent magical powers, take on responsibility and at the same time face loss, separation and death.

In a similar vein, Bennett's story traces the Queen's internal development as a result of her reading. After Norman is suddenly removed, Bennett's narrator observes how little the Queen seems troubled. The narrator comments on how typical it was for the Queen's courtiers to spare her any 'distress or even fellow feeling' by keeping anything likely to arouse such feelings from her. Much later when she meets Norman again, she is aware of his upset. The narrator comments she then knows more about others' feelings, and can put herself in someone else's place. She moves from feeling entitled not to be concerned about others, to noticing other people's feelings and to feel concern for them.

Without Norman with whom to discuss her reading, the Queen starts to make copious notes including observations about herself and others. She notes a recommendation that 'one recipe for happiness is to have no sense of entitlement', and adds her comment that 'this is not a lesson I have ever been in a position to learn'. Thinking about approaching the end of her life she concludes that, unlike the authors she reads, she has had no voice of her own. She despairs of her reading in observing to herself 'You don't put your life into your books. You find it there'. She determines to try to write and publish her observations. She thus becomes able to observe herself whilst being herself, most evident in her abdication speech which illustrates her capacity to observe her part in corruption and cover up, and wish to make reparation.

The therapeutic aspects of reading are now well recognised and acknowledged by the UK's National Institute for Health and Clinical Excellence in its guidelines about bibliotherapy. Little has appeared in psychoanalytic litera-ture about the therapeutic processes in reading. Exceptionally, Christopher Bollas (1978) has written about the search for transformative experiences through reading. He refers specifically to experiences of 'deep subjective rapport between reader and text', which may be evoked from a few words or an entire piece of literature, or some other art form. He argues that such aes-thetic experiences are recollections of our earliest experiences of maternal care, when this kind of communion with mother gives the infant the experience of mother as a 'transformational object'. Bollas refers to the transformational promise as 'where the unintegrations of self find integration through the form provided by the transformational object' (p. 385). This transformation is similar to the holding which Bick (1968) described when the mother provides the infant with a sense of a psychic 'skin' holding together all the infant's disparate feelings and experiences.

The transformative shift from paranoid-schizoid to depressive functioning that Bennett is illustrating in reading can also be seen in therapy in the development which enables therapists to move from holding to containing (Caper, 1999), or patient-centred to therapist-centred (Steiner, 1993) interpretations, discussed in Chapter 1. This movement facilitates the patient in disentangling him or herself from projections which distort the truth. Bennett well illustrates this kind of therapeutic transformation in the Queen's abdication speech in the way she was able to acknowledge painful truths about herself.

Bernardine Bishop (2001) reveals Shakespeare commenting on this therapeutic process in his somewhat unusual epilogue to *The Tempest* when Prospero invites the audience to 'draw near' and asks for our help in leaving the island saying:

> Let me not ... dwell
> In this bare island by your spell.
> But release me from my bands
> With the help of your good hands ...
> As you from crimes would pardoned be
> Let your indulgence set me free.
>   (Folger Shakespeare Library, p. 170)

At the play's end I see Prospero pleading not to be left with our projections. He tells us we can set him free by withdrawing our projections, and taking responsibility for our own guilt and wish for forgiveness. If Bennett succeeds, neither should we leave the Queen seeking redemption through analysis and reflection, but engage ourselves in reflecting on our own collusion in narcissistic entitlement, omnipotence and corruption.

My Epilogue

For reading groups in prisons there is mounting evidence about the value of reading in enhancing personal growth and providing substantial benefits for rehabilitation. One aspect repeatedly cited is the gain in prisoners' capacities for empathy with others. Despite such evidence, the UK government attempted to restrict prisoners' access to books. Key literary figures including Bennett protested. *The Uncommon Reader* demonstrates how Bennett understands the importance of reading, and how passionately he must have felt about the protest. Perhaps his understanding of infantile narcissism meant he was not surprised by what the government tried to do.

References

Bennett, A. (2006). *The Uncommon Reader.* London: Faber and Faber.

Bick, E. (1968). The experience of skin in early object relations. In E. Bott-Spillius E. (Ed.) *Melanie Klein To-day, Volume 1.* London: Routledge.

Bishop, B. (2001). Lear and Prospero: From the projective to the introjective mode. *British Journal of Psychotherapy*, 17 (4), 505–17.

Bollas, C. (1978). The aesthetic moment and the search for transformation. *The Annual of Psychoanalysis*, 6, 385–94.

Caper, R. (1999). *A Mind of One's Own.* London: Routledge.

Freud, S. (1914). On narcissism: An introduction. In J. Strachey, A. Freud, A. Strachey & A. Tyson (Eds) *The Standard Edition of the Complete Psychological Works of Sigmund Freud. Volume XIV* (pp. 67–102). London: Hogarth Press.

Shakespeare, W. *The Tempest.* Mowat, B., Werstine, P., Poston, M. & Niles, R. (Eds) Folger Shakespeare Library. Washington, DC: Folger Shakespeare Library. https://shakespeare.folger.edu/shakespeares-works/the-tempest/act-5-epilogue/

Tuckett, D., & Taffler, R. (2008). Phantastic Objects and the Financial Market's Sense of Reality: A Psychoanalytic Contribution to the Understanding of Stock Market Instability. *International Journal of Psychoanalysis*, 89, 389–412.

Chapter 12

Sexual Identity

Colm Toibin's novel *Nora Webster* (2014) took him thirteen years to write during which he completed several other novels including *Brooklyn* which won the Costa Book Award. He explained he struggled writing *Nora Webster* because it was so closely based on his personal experience of loss and grief. He was twelve when his father died. Toibin recalled he felt numb and unable to put any feelings into words, but clearly he was a most observant young fellow. This novel is a beautifully written account of a woman's emotional experience following her husband's traumatic death, and being left with two young boys and two older girls. It is the interiority of Nora's experience and the depth of understanding of her grief that makes this a remarkable book, a testimony to Toibin's empathy. As a youth he may not have had words but as an adult he eloquently conveys his mother's experience of bereavement. This novel led me to thinking about mourning and sexual identity.

Nora struggles with mourning. She abandons her two boys during her husband Maurice's excruciating dying in hospital. She arranged for the boys to stay with her aunt and made no contact with them for over two months. Her loss was unbearable, she projectively evoked aspects of this loss in her boys who were distressed not to hear from her. After Maurice's death, faced with limited finance she needs to find some work in order to make ends meet. She can only manage by putting her grief aside. She discourages any discussion of her own or the children's feelings, a form of splitting sometimes necessary in order to survive. During her trials to establish a secure financial footing she nevertheless reflects on the impact of the loss of Maurice on herself and her children. She comes to appreciate the effect on the boys of her abandonment of them during Maurice's dying. She revisits the death of her father when she was in her teens, and later the death of her mother with whom she had a poor relationship. These earlier, probably unmourned, deaths give some indications of the source of her difficulties in mourning Maurice.

Three years later Nora has made a secure life for her family. As she begins decorating a room of her own, she experiences the full impact of her grief.

DOI: 10.4324/9781003319719-17

She collapses and is nursed to recovery by her aunt. In a state of physical and emotional exhaustion, Nora hallucinates Maurice alive and talking to her. Nora is troubled by Maurice's insistence that there was now 'one other'. He could not be reassured when she told him there was no-one else. Nora tells her aunt about Maurice remonstrating about the one other. Her aunt assures her the conversation was a dream. The one other remains an enigma. I see the one other as Nora herself whose journey through grief is leading to a transformation in her identity, she is discovering a mind of her own. Pursuing this line of thought I revisited Jean White's psychoanalytic commentary on Homer's Odyssey (2009). White traces Odysseus' transformation during perilous adventures on his epic journey from Troy back to his home in Ithaca. She draws on contemporary developments in psychoanalytic theory to elucidate her understanding of the transformation in Odysseus' identity. White discusses how Odysseus' narrow escapes involve him symbolically shedding different aspects of his identity, until finally he arrives home unrecognisable, looking like a beggar and utterly alone. An example of this shedding is when Odysseus slays the one-eyed monster Cyclops, who has captured him and devoured some of his men. White, citing Bion, interprets this episode symbolically as Odysseus shedding a monocular perspective and gaining a capacity to view the same thing from multiple 'vertices'.

Odysseus' journey into the unknown realms of the various islands includes visiting Hades, where he meets his mother who died whilst he was away. He eventually loses all of his men with whom he started his journey; they are either slaughtered or ship-wrecked. White sees Odysseus' symbolic aloneness 'as an integral aspect of human evolution'. She quotes Christopher Bollas who warns that personal growth, accomplished by shedding aspects of identity, means entering unknown realms and bearing the aloneness of inhabiting a mind of one's own. White does not explore Odysseus' mourning for his mother or his lost comrades, or the part mourning might have contributed in the development in his identity. I see such transformation enabled by mourning. I understand shedding aspects of identity and developing a capacity for aloneness are achieved as a result of mourning one's separateness and omnipotence, and thereby disentangling oneself from mutual projective identifications with others. Caper (1999) describes this process as developing a mind of one's own; and discusses the consequent aloneness quoting Bion (1963) who, in *Elements of Psychoanalysis*, emphasised the need for bearing a sense of isolation within an intimate relationship.

Nora's transformation is exemplified in the way she quite literally finds a voice of her own. It seems during her marriage to Maurice she was often silent, over-awed by his views. After his death she begins to speak up about local politics to Maurice's brother who, she feels pleased to notice, is shocked. She challenges the headmaster of the school where Maurice taught. The headmaster intends to treat her youngest son in a way she feels unjust, and which the headmaster would not have pursued whilst Maurice was alive. The headmaster will not budge. She speaks to the other teachers and threatens to arrange a boycott for 'Justice' outside the school. She succeeds in making the headmaster climb down. She reveals her vocal talent, and comes to enjoy developing her singing, which she had previously neglected out of resentment against her mother who was an accomplished vocalist. She discovers a love of classical music, something Maurice would not have shared or perhaps even condoned; and she imagines a professional life in music which she might have developed had she not married.

In these examples of Nora finding her own voice, she is disentangling herself from disabling projections with which she became identified. When she gives voice to her political thoughts in male company, she retrieves some of her own capacities which were projectively attributed to Maurice; and in becoming more separate from him she begins to observe his misogyny and is then less influenced by his misogynistic projections. Hence, she is more able to be in touch with and use her aggression in rebutting the headmaster's misogynistically licensed ill-treatment of her youngest son. She sees that the headmaster would not have attempted this when Maurice was alive, but because she is a woman he thinks he can get away with it. When Nora nurtures and enjoys her gift for singing, she has freed herself from being influenced by a negative identification with her mother which prevented her pursuing her own singing talents.

A key aria which inspires Nora's newfound interest in classical music is from Dvorak's opera *Rusalka*, a song of love sung by the water nymph heroine about a human prince she has seen on the shore. The nymph gains permission to leave her watery domain to become human and pursue the prince, on condition that she forfeits her power of speech. If she doesn't find love, she will be damned and the man she loves will die. Rusalka is about to marry the prince when she overhears him expressing his love for another woman. The prince dies, Rusalka is alone, sings her final aria and disappears back into the water. The story of the opera bears a striking resonance with Nora's silence during her marriage, and discovery of her voice following Maurice's death. This resonance is probably no mere coincidence because Toibin admits to deriving inspiration from classical music. I see the stories of these liaisons, Nora's and Rusalka's, as illustrations of projectively merged relationships which may try to escape the aloneness of trying to inhabit a mind of one's own. I think this kind of relationship, especially for women, may be particularly disabling because of our deeply entrenched misogynistic society. The mutual identifications involved can mean becoming enmeshed in negative projective identifications of womanhood and femininity. As a gay man I have experienced and seen misogyny also affecting gay men and their relationships; for example, in being taunted by 'straight' men and women for being like a girl or a 'cissy', and in the fear of being exposed as not a proper man. I have also observed how members of the gay community, including myself, can often revile others who are camp or effeminate. By contrast Toibin, who is gay, has a marvellous capacity evident in his writings, to identify with women's experiences.

A novel that pursues the theme of misogyny and some of its worst effects on women is by the celebrated Australian writer Kate Grenville. *Dark Places* (1994) tells the story of a Victorian patriarch and has been praised for its chilling character study of a sexual monster. In interviews about her writing, Grenville has acknowledged her gratitude for having had a psychoanalysis. She said she could only have written *Dark Places* because she recognised her own misogyny. Grenville's insight illustrates another difficulty in the shedding of misogynistic identifications; whatever our gender we need to recognise our own misogyny. Projective identification takes hold by projectively evoking aspects of the self which have particular affinity with the projections (Brenman Pick, 1985). Projections of misogyny will find hooks in the recipient's misogyny.

In their introduction to *Sexualities: Contemporary Psychoanalytic Perspectives* (2015) Alexandra Lemma and Paul Lynch return to Freud's view that we are all bisexual. This insight had been overlooked by Freud's followers since he first wrote about it at the beginning of the last century. Moreover, some psychoanalysts have expressed highly prejudiced positions about homosexuality and most of the psychoanalytic literature shows an absence of any reference to homoerotic counter-transference. Acknowledging an innate bisexuality implies recognising a fluid sexual identity irrespective of one's biological gender, and a capacity to love as well as hate men and women, and to love and hate one's own masculine and feminine qualities. The disturbance in society as the trans community finds its voice, is indicative of the disturbance caused by a loosening and even rejection of biologically assigned genders of male and female, and of the rigid binary categories of sexual identity. If we can bear the disturbance, the voices of trans people bring an opportunity for us all to reflect on our fluid, ambiguous sexual identities often hidden in fears and prejudices, without too quickly foreclosing such reflection by denial or resort to surgical interventions (Patterson, 2018). In the spirit of inhabiting a mind of one's own and bearing aloneness, we could try shedding biologically and socially assigned sexual identities. Such journeys exploring and shedding the certainties of our sexual identities mean mourning the losses of those certainties, and recognising the hatred for aspects of our identities which may have been disowned, split off and projectively evoked in others who have suffered our hatred in the form of external or internalised misogyny and homophobia.

References

Bion, W.R. (1963). *Elements of Psychoanalysis*. London: Basic Books.

Brenman Pick, I. (1985). Working through in the countertransference. *International Journal of Psychoanalysis*, 66, 157–66.

Caper, R. (1999). *A Mind of One's Own*. London: Routledge.

Grenville, K. (1994). *Dark Places*. London: Picador.

Lemma, A. & Lynch, P. (Eds) (2015). *Sexualities: Contemporary Psychoanalytic Perspectives*. London: Routledge.

Patterson, T. (2018). Unconscious homophobia and the rise of the transgender movement. *Psychodynamic Practice, 24* (1), 56–9.

Toibin, C. (2014). *Nora Webster*. London: Penguin

White, J. (2009). The Odyssey: Contemporary psychoanalytic perspectives. *British Journal of Psychotherapy, 25* (4), 493–505.

Some Kleinian Concepts

This is a short summary for readers unfamiliar with Kleinian ideas. For an introduction to Klein I recommend *Introduction to the Work of Melanie Klein* (1988) by Hanna Segal.

Internal Objects

Klein, who worked therapeutically with young children as well as adults, elucidated how from early life we form identifications with others who in the unconscious are portrayed as living in an internal world inside our bodies, which she described as internal objects. Klein described how these identifications vary according to our states of mind and emotional resources, and the associated anxieties and defences. She formulated two main 'positions' which recur throughout life, a 'paranoid-schizoid' and a 'depressive position'.

The Paranoid-Schizoid Position

The paranoid-schizoid position was elaborated for the first time in Klein's 'Notes on some schizoid mechanisms' (Klein, 1946). Klein outlined this position as a set of persecutory fears and defences, which are aspects of early infantile mental life to which we return throughout the life cycle, especially when we are faced with adversity. In these states of mind we need to resort to omnipotent phantasy that offers absolute certainty, an all or nothing, black or white view of our world, in which for example following a catastrophe like '9/11' others are 'either with us or against us'. Under extreme duress, we may have no capacity for tolerating not knowing or uncertainty, because we do not have the emotional resources or support to bear more complex, ambivalent and realistic views of ourselves and others. In paranoid-schizoid states of mind, our identifications with others are likely to result in internal objects which are possessed and controlled by projective identification to deny separateness and loss (Caper, 1999).

The Depressive Position

It was in Klein's study of mourning (1940) that she formulated the depressive position, following her understanding of the kind of the identifications and internalisations that result from successful mourning. Mourning means being able to acknowledge our hatred as well as love for the lost loved one, the loved one's loving and hating aspects, our own and other's limitations, the limits of life itself and our separateness. In the unconscious the mourner feels responsible for the loss of the loved one because of his or her ambivalence and destructiveness. It is the mourner's guilt and remorse that fuels reparation and restoration of the loved one in the internal world.

Early in life, it is the mother or primary carer who nurtures the infant's and child's capacities to bear loss and separation through her receptiveness and containment of projected unbearable states of mind. If all proceeds well, the achievement of the depressive position means there is less need of splitting and projection, and a capacity to bear separateness and acknowledge the freedom of others. Consequently, there are changes in the kinds of identification with and internalisation of others in our internal world. These changes come about initially through the love, care and containment of our primary carers, and later of our loved ones, whereby we manage to integrate loving and hating qualities into our identity, and loved and hated qualities into our view of others. Our internal world is then inhabited with representations of others as internal objects in a way which recognises their freedom and separateness (Caper, 1999).

The capacity to mourn represents a huge developmental achievement which throughout life requires considerable emotional strength and resources, which may not always be available. Under severe stress and adversity our capacities may be diminished and we may slip into paranoid-schizoid states of mind.

Psychoanalytic Studies of Psychosis which Informed My Work

In Freud's (1895) early thoughts from his discussions about a woman suffering from psychotic episodes he noted that there was 'a clearsighted and calm observer sat, as she put it, in a corner of her brain and looked on at all the mad business' (p. 26). Later, in his study of the memoirs of Schreber, a judge who suffered from psychosis, Freud (1911) understood projection and reparative aspects in psychotic symptoms. He understood Schreber's delusion about the end of the world as a projection of an internal catastrophe that had already happened, a catastrophe involving the destruction of Schreber's mind when he suffered a psychotic breakdown. Freud saw Schreber's delusions as 'an attempt at recovery, a process of reconstruction' (1911, p. 71). Despite achieving some success with psychotic patients Freud remained pessimistic about psychoanalytic treatment of psychosis. He thought people suffering from psychosis were turning away from reality to narcissism and hence were unable to establish a transference relationship (Rosenfeld, 1987, p. 282). Some of Freud's psychoanalytic colleagues and later generations of analysts explored different ways of working with psychotic patients, though often making considerable changes to traditional psychoanalytic technique (see Rosenfeld's summary, 1987, p. 281–311).

Klein worked with some children suffering from psychosis. She concluded that the fixation points in the psychoses went back to early childhood. She described certain anxieties of the infant and child as psychotic, because of the resemblance of these anxieties to those of adult psychotic patients. In particular she described 'persecutory anxieties' about fears of survival of the self, occurring in paranoid states, and 'depressive anxieties' about concerns for the survival of others as well as the self, occurring in depressive psychoses. Klein's (1946) discoveries about projective identification significantly influenced understanding about narcissism and the treatment of psychosis. In particular Klein drew attention to an underlying depression (1960) and loneliness (1963) in people suffering from schizophrenia which were often not apparent because of the use of splitting and projective identification.

Several of Klein's closest colleagues, Hanna Segal, Wilfrid Bion and Herbert Rosenfeld, who were to become leading exponents of her ideas, began working with psychotic patients without altering the psychoanalytic technique. A central concept in developments by these three pioneers was projective identification and the pathological use of this mechanism which is characteristic of psychotic patients. Segal (1957) showed how the concrete thinking typical of schizophrenic patients, reflects the excessive use of projective identification. The boundary between self and others becomes so obscured by projection that it is not possible to distinguish between the object and the symbol which represents it. The illustration she gave was of a patient who refused to play the violin saying that he did not want to masturbate in public. Segal called this a 'symbolic equation' in which the symbol is concretely equated with the object. Segal (1956) reported how schizophrenic patients unable to manage depressive anxieties could projectively evoke these feelings in the analyst. Hinshelwood (1989, p. 411) suggested that Freud's pessimism about treating psychotic patients may have reflected such a projective process in which Freud was affected by his patients' underlying depression.

Bion (1957) understood that psychotic patients' hatred of reality meant they attempted to destroy their perceptual functions in an omnipotent phantasy of splitting them into minute particles, and projecting these into external objects which became what he called 'bizarre objects', because such objects in phantasy included these particles. For example, if a patient projects an auditory function into a television, it may be experienced as listening to the patient. He wrote 'Such is the dominance of this phantasy, but a fact to the patient, who acts as if his perceptual apparatus could be split into minute fragments and projected into his objects' (p. 64). Bion pointed out omnipotent phantasy was part of a psychotic personality, and its dominance obscured a non-psychotic personality in which the ego retains contact with reality. Bion maintained there is a psychotic and non psychotic personality within everyone. In someone suffering from psychosis the psychotic personality is dominant and is distinguished by omnipotent phantasy, and reliance on projective identification. In contrast, the non-psychotic personality uses repression, keeping aspects of oneself unconscious without needing to split them off and in phantasy project those aspects into others. Unlike Freud, Bion and his Kleinian colleagues were optimistic about therapy for those suffering from psychosis. Their understanding of projective identification and omnipotent phantasy brought hope. Moreover they found that people suffering from psychosis could be successfully treated psychoanalytically.

Rosenfeld (1987) made intensive studies of narcissism and its relationship with psychosis. In working with psychotic patients he described a 'transference psychosis', which develops through an omnipotent use of projective identification into the analyst. It is the omnipotent quality of the projective identification which leads to narcissism, and distinguishes it from projective identification used in ordinary development. Rosenfeld described how omnipotent narcissistic parts of the self can link up with psychotic parts of the personality. Like Bion he emphasized the importance of recognising a sane or healthy part that co-exists even within the most flagrantly deluded patient. Rosenfeld also noted that there may be different degrees of disturbance within the psychotic parts of the personality.

Rosenfeld explained that a negative therapeutic reaction may at times be caused by severe mental pain as a result of insight developing in the sane part of the personality, which cannot bear the pain. Negative therapeutic reactions refer to times in therapy when there is a moment or period of useful and important contact between patient and therapist which is followed by a backward, regressive, sometimes destructive movement. Rosenfeld (1981, p. 171) wrote the 'most frequent negative therapeutic reactions occur when the saner more object related parts of the personality appear openly in the transference situation. This almost immediately mobilises violent opposition of the psychotic omnipotent structure of the patient's personality which feels threatened in its position of absolute power and domination of the patient.'

Rosenfeld distinguishes between a 'libidinal' narcissism and a 'destructive' narcissism. In the libidinal narcissism it is the positive aspects of the personality which are idealized whereas in destructive narcissism it is the negative or bad aspects which are idealized. Destructive narcissism is often hard to recognise because it can operate as a silent, deadly and deadening force within the personality, which can hypnotize and paralyze the sane or healthy parts, or it may be disguised and present itself in benevolent and kindly ways. When analytic work reveals the destructive aspects, they sometimes appear in dreams represented by a mafia gang which terrorizes and holds to ransom the sane parts of the personality. Destructive narcissism has a hatred of recognising need and the dependent parts of the personality. When the destructive narcissism joins up with psychotic parts of the personality, it offers promises of a delusional pain-free state where any sadistic pleasure can be enjoyed and where there is no need for anyone.

Rosenfeld drew attention to confusional states and confusional anxieties, particularly in people suffering from schizophrenia. The dominance of projective identification means there may be a confusion of what is good and bad. Further extreme splitting may follow to relieve these anxieties, so it may be preferable to feel all bad than to be in any doubt about it. Rosenfeld described examples of negative counter-transference reactions resulting from analysts confusing different parts of the patient, interpreting patient's material as attacks from the psychotic personality. Whereas, Rosenfeld argued that what were seen as attacks were a sane part of the patient trying to communicate with the analyst.

The analysis of people suffering from psychosis was relatively short-lived. Few analysts continue to work in the public health institutions. In the UK, units specially devoted to psychoanalytic work with psychotic patients have been closed down (Lucas, 1992). Among later analysts and others working with a psychoanalytic orientation who continued to take an interest in this field, Sohn (1985) described the narcissistic organization as an 'identificate', and emphasized the omnipotence of the identification such that the psychotic personality is very intolerant of there being any sense of other parts of the self. He mentions the particular quality of untrustworthiness experienced in the counter-transference. He explained when in contact with this kind of patient the analyst is led to feel all his psychoanalytic expertise is worthless.

A sense of untrustworthiness is echoed by John Steiner's view of destructive narcissism as a pathological organization of defences, or as he later describes them 'psychic retreats', which defend against the fragmentation of the paranoid-schizoid position or the depressive anxieties of the depressive position. Britton (1998) sees these pathological organizations as a defence against madness of the paranoid-schizoid position or against reality of the depressive position. Hinshelwood (1989) describes the origins of this concept of a structured defensive organization which has emerged in post Kleinian work, as a development from Freud's (1911) formulations about the Schreber case, in which he understood the defensive structure followed a psychotic breakdown.

Steiner's concept of pathological organizations integrates the concepts of destructive narcissism, psychotic parts of the personality and later post Kleinian work on defensive organizations. Steiner arrives at this integration in the following way:

'If we assume that a primitive destructive part of the self exists in all individuals, an important determinant of the outcome will be the way this destructiveness is dealt with by the remaining parts of the personality. In psychotic patients this destructive part of the self dominates the personality, destroying and immobilizing the healthy parts. In the normal individual the destructive part is less split off so that it can to a greater extent be contained and neutralized by the healthy parts of the personality. There remains an intermediate situation in which the balance is more even, which results clinically in borderline and narcissistic states. Here the destructive part of the self cannot completely ignore the healthy parts and is forced to take account of them and enter into a liaison with them'.
(Steiner, 1982, p. 242)

Steiner notes that although it may appear the sane parts are a victim of the psychotic parts, the sane parts may be in collusion with the psychotic parts. In other words it is important to keep an open mind about the relationship between these different parts of the personality.

Lucas (1992) described some shocking examples of how active, and yet how well concealed the psychotic parts may be, and how seriously they may put the life of the patient at risk. Developing the theme of untrustworthiness, he wrote of the importance of helping staff not to be taken in by the apparent plausibility of the psychotic part, but to try to tune into the 'psychotic wave-length' (1993) of the patient. For example, he described how a patient's suicidal state which seemed to arise out of hopelessness and despair, in fact masked a murderous attack by the psychotic personality in reaction against the non-psychotic personality engaging in the therapy. On another occasion it was because a member of staff recognized the covert participation of the psychotic personality that a patient, who otherwise claimed she was taking care of herself, was rescued from a suicidal attempt. Lucas described a dream of a schizophrenic patient which, despite a psychotic breakdown, indicated the continued existence of the non-psychotic personality. In the dream the whole world had been destroyed by a nuclear holocaust, but on a remote outer planet there were signs of surviving life (Lucas, 1992, p. 75). This dream also illustrates Freud's view of an internal disaster in a psychotic breakdown.

Michael Sinason (1993) and Joscelyn Richards (1999), who established a successful psychotherapy service in London for psychotic patients, go so far as to postulate the existence of two independent minds inhabiting the same body, a sane one and a psychotic one which they call the 'co-habitee'. They reject the notion of a unitary ego trying to manage sane and psychotic parts in therapy. Instead they see their goal as helping the patient to better understand and manage the disturbed co-habiting self. They are particularly cautious in their technique not to undermine the sane self by confusing it with the psychotic self, or to inflame the psychotic co-habitee by being critical, deni-gratory or rejecting of it. They discuss their detailed tracking within sessions of the moment-by-moment fluctuations of the psychotic and non-psychotic personalities, and ways of talking to their patients about these processes. Their careful attention to monitoring their own 'cohabitee' responses to the patient is a reminder of the therapist's need to be alert to psychotic parts of the therapist's personality being evoked in the counter-transference.

References

Bion, W.R. (1957). Differentiation of the psychotic from the non-psychotic personal-ities. *International Journal of Psycho-Analysis*, *38*, 266–75.

Britton, R. (1998). *Belief and Imagination*. London: Routledge.

Caper, R. (1999). *A Mind of One's Own*. London: Routledge.

Freud, S. (1911). Psychoanalytical notes on an autobiographical account of a case of paranoia. *The Standard Edition of the Complete Psychological Works of Sigmund Freud* (Dementia Paranoides) XII (pp. 1–82). London: Hogarth Press.

Freud, S. & Breuer, J. (1895). *Studies in Hysteria*. London: Pengui

Hinshelwood, R. (1989). *A Dictionary of Kleinian Thought*. London: Free Association.

Klein. M. (1940). Mourning and its Relation to Manic-Depressive States. *International Journal of Psychoanalysis*, *21*, 125–53.

Klein, M. (1946). Notes on some schizoid mechanisms. *International Journal of Psychoanalysis*, *27*, 99–110.

Klein, M. (1960). Symposium on 'Depressive Illness' – V. A Note on Depression in the Schizophrenic. *International Journal of Psychoanalysis*, *41*, 509–11.

Klein, M. (1963). On the sense of loneliness. In *The Writings of Melanie Klein Volume III*. London: Hogarth.

Lucas, R.N. (1992). The psychotic personality: a psychoanalytical theory and its application in clinical practice. *Psychoanalytic Psychotherapy*, *7* (1), 3– 17.

Rosenfeld, H. (1981). On the psychopathology and treatment of psychotic patients (historical and comparative reflections). In J. Grotestein (Ed.) *Do I Dare Disturb the Universe?* London: Karnac.

Rosenfeld, H. (1987). *Impasse and Interpretation*. London: Tavistock.

Richards, J. (1999). The concept of internal co-habitation. In S. Johnson & S. Ruszcynski (Eds) *Psychoanalytic Psychotherapy in the Independent Tradition*. London: Karnac.

Segal, H. (1956). Depression in the schizophrenic. In E. Bott Spillius (Ed.) (1988). *Melanie Klein Today Volume 1*. London: Routledge.

Segal, H. (1957). Notes on symbol formation. In E. Bott Spillius (Ed.) (1988). *Melanie Klein Today Volume 1*. London: Routledge.

Sinason, M. (1993). Who is the mad voice inside? *Psychoanalytic Psychotherapy*, *7* (3), 207–21.

Sohn, L. (1985). Narcissistic organization, projective identification and the formation of the identificate. In E. Bott Spillius (Ed.) (1988). *Melanie Klein Today Volume 1*. London: Routledge.

Steiner, J. (1982). Perverse relationships between parts of the self: A clinical illustration. *International Journal of Psychoanalysis*, *63*, 241–51.

Index